D1142749

★ ★ ★ YOUR ★ ★ ★ PERSONAL TRAINER

Dr. Kathy Fulcher & Pat Fox

metro

The Sheffield College

Hillsborough LRC
☎ 0114 2602254

ACC No.   111445925

Class   Loan Category
613.7   L

This edition first published in Great Britain in 2002
by Metro Publishing Limited, 3 Bramber Court,
2 Bramber Road, London W14 9PB

All rights reserved: no part of this publication may be
reproduced, stored in a retrieval system, or transmitted in
any form or by any means, electronic, mechanical,
photocopying or otherwise, without the prior written
consent of the publisher.

Text © 2002 Kathy Fulcher and Pat Fox
Illustrations by Richard Burgess
Illustrations © 2002 Metro Publishing

Kathy Fulcher and Pat Fox are hereby identified as the
authors of this work in accordance with Section 77 of the
Copyright, Designs and Patents Act 1988.

The training programmes in this book have been devised
with safety in mind. The authors and publisher cannot be
held liable for injury sustained during training.

British Library Cataloguing in Publication Data.
A CIP record of this book is available on request
from the British Library.

ISBN 1 84358 002 0

10 9 8 7 6 5 4 3 2 1

Typeset in 9/12 Leawood Book
Printed and Bound in Great Britain by CPD (Wales)

Contents

ACKNOWLEDGEMENTS

The Cooper 12-minute test (page 16); 1½-mile run test (page 16); Estimated Maximal VO$_2$ (page 17) all taken from R. V. Hockey, *Physical Fitness: The Pathway to Healthful Living*, 1993, 7th edition, reproduced by permission of The McGraw-Hill companies, USA.

Rotator Cuff exercises (pages 164–6) reprinted by kind permission of Physio Tools Ltd, UK.

Maximal Oxygen Consumption table (pages 18–19), based on norms from *The Physical Fitness Specialist Manual*, The Cooper Institute for Aerobic Research, Dallas, Texas, revised 1998; used with permission.

Carbohydrate and Energy Expenditure tables (pages 248-51) taken from F. I. Katch and W. D. McCardle, *Introduction to Nutrition, Exercise and Health*, 1993, 4th edition, reprinted by kind permission of Williams & Wilkins, Maryland, USA.

I would like to acknowledge all those coaches, athletes and scientists I have worked with over the years – I have learned from all of you. In particular, I would like to dedicate this book to my parents, Ida and Henry Fox, both of whom taught me the value of sport and persistence; to Tony Foster who taught me to never give up in the face of adversity; and, finally, to the face of adversity, camaraderie and lifelong friendship, the boys of 249b.

Pat Fox

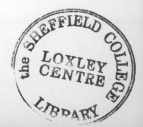

Introduction

Welcome to *Your Personal Trainer* – a book that will help you to get ready for your chosen sport, no matter at what level you wish to take part.

When considering different sports and making a choice of sport, it is important to remember that excellence in sports depends on a number of factors. For some sports, genetics and the body shape or structure with which you are born are important: top marathon runners or gymnasts are typical examples of individuals who have naturally selected a sport because of their body type. Many other sports are more dependent on training and technique, and anyone who follows a well-structured and appropriate training programme should do well.

Bearing these considerations in mind, and even if only a few will progress to élite levels, anyone starting a sport can expect to progress to a very reasonable competitive level if they work at it. This is where *Your Personal Trainer* fits in and is set to become your training companion. The aim of all sports training is to improve fitness and skills, and to develop training programmes that are safe and effective. To do this properly, an understanding of the metabolic and physiological demands of the sport is needed. All sports require combinations of strength, speed, endurance, agility and flexibility to varying degrees. What is important is how these elements are all integrated to enhance the skills of the sport in question. Other factors to be taken into account in your training programme are the stage of a season, nutrition, the importance of avoiding injuries, your health status, and the nature and role of other team players. All this information is given in a concise and easily understandable way for each of the sports covered in this book.

The first few chapters explain the fundamentals that you need to know and give you the tools to find out more about your own health and fitness level. Whether you are already quite fit or a complete beginner, it is important to assess your starting level, both to give you a benchmark from which to chart your progress and to ensure that you approach your training safely. These chapters lead you through the jungle of training terminology to give you a better understanding of the basic principles of training.

Resistance training has a role to play in many sports, and Chapter 5, dedicated to this area of training, goes into detail on the different modes of resistance training as well as the different ways to structure resistance-training programmes. If you are not already familiar with weight-training exercises (which we do not describe in detail), it is safest and most beneficial to ask for a demonstration and one-to-one tuition at a gym by a qualified instructor, either with free weights or machines.

The 15 sports-specific sections explain the structure of each sport, the energy systems involved in playing it, the muscles used and the sport's fundamentals, as well as outlining the ideal player profile. Training programmes start at the beginner (entry) level, going through a transition stage, which allows you to assess whether you are ready to move up to a more advanced and, of course, more demanding training programme.

The training programmes given for each of the sports take you through all the preparation stages, right up to the competitive season. They will help you to develop desirable fitness levels and to ally them to sports skills such that, as individuals and teams, you can improve and progress. They do not cover training during the competitive season. Competitive seasons and match or race schedules vary considerably between sports and levels of competitions, and it is therefore impossible to include them within the scope of this book. However, the understanding that you will gain from this book of the practicalities of training should give you the confidence to put this part of your training programme together yourself.

The final chapters give details on healthy eating for sport and explain how to avoid injury, so that your sports participation will be long and enjoyable.

Whatever your sport and whatever your level, we hope that this book will give you the information you need to train hard, train well and have fun.

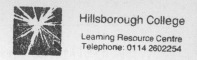

Hillsborough College

Learning Resource Centre
Telephone: 0114 2602254

CHAPTER 1

The Nuts and Bolts

THE VALUE OF SPORTING ACTIVITY

Most sporting activities have a good, general effect on the body. The training programmes in this book aim to ensure that any benefit is safely achieved. But remember you need to be fairly fit before you can begin. Or, at the very least, start working on getting fitter the moment you begin your sport. Just playing or doing your sport will not get you fit unless you are at a very basic level.

Of course, there are other benefits such as enjoying being part of a team, having fun, relief of muscular pain and so on. But for now your primary goal is physical fitness.

THE WHYS AND WHEREFORES OF TRAINING

First, you need to get used to the general ideas and principles of the basic training programme. These include:

- why you need warm-up and cool-down periods
- what terms such as 'frequency', 'duration' and 'intensity' mean
- understanding the types of energy systems involved
- how to use your heart rate to assess and monitor the way you train (this is explained in Chapter 4)
- making a yearly training plan – where it all fits together and how to plan for your sport (this is explained in Chapter 3).

1

Why do you need to warm up?

To get the most out of your training session, match, game or race you must first warm up. The main effect of a warm-up is to raise body temperature including, of course, muscle temperature. It also prepares you for more strenuous exercise by speeding up your heart rate and increasing metabolic rate so that energy is released faster.

When you rest, or at any time when you are not particularly active, not only is your blood circulating around your body, but a good deal of it is busy in your digestive system. An active warm-up will divert some of the blood supply to the active muscles so that fuel and oxygen get to them more quickly. A warm-up also reduces the risk of placing unnecessary stress on your heart. Other warm-up benefits include:

- making your muscles more flexible, or elastic, so that they are less prone to strains or tears
- getting you mentally ready for the exercise to follow
- increasing alertness
- speeding up the nerve impulses to your muscles and the speed at which messages travel from your brain to your muscle
- reducing muscle stiffness after exercise.

What does a warm-up involve?

A warm-up should begin very gently with some low-intensity aerobic exercise that is gradually increased. This can be brisk walking, jogging (outdoors or on the spot), easy cycling or, if you are about to do a swimming session, a few gentle lengths of an easy stroke. Almost any activity will do (even dancing) as long as it starts off gently. This should last 5-10 minutes and should be followed by stretching.

The stretching you do in your warm-up is not the main bulk of your flexibility work. You will gain a lot more from stretching if you do it *after* your main exercise or training session when your body is well warmed up and you will see a greater range of movement. Stretching is covered in much greater detail in Chapter 6.

The final part of the warm-up depends on your sport. For sports such as football, rugby and hockey you should include some fast bursts: not flat-out sprints, but stride-outs. If you are about to play a game, follow this with some passing practice and drills. For sports such as tennis, squash, table tennis, volleyball and basketball the pre-game warm-up should include some court shuttle runs, not flat-out sprints, followed by some sport-specific drills or a knock-up.

Why do you need to cool down?

After a training session, match or game, spend some time letting the body cool down gradually. You need to allow the blood to be re-routed from the muscles to the rest of your body to restore the balance. If you stop suddenly after exercise with no gradual cooling or slowing down, the short delay in re-routing the blood can make you feel dizzy. Also, rather like a car engine producing exhaust fumes, burning fuel in the body creates waste products in the muscles during exercise and these need to be cleared away from the muscles after the exercise. These unwanted products can cause muscle soreness and stiffness after exercise. Slowing down gradually allows time for your system to clear them out and should reduce stiffness when accompanied by stretching.

How do I cool down?

The cool-down is very similar to the warm-up, but in reverse. Now you gradually decrease the intensity of your exercise. As for the warm-up, do 5-10 minutes of any form of gentle aerobic activity. Follow this with some stretching exercises. Focus particularly on the muscles you have used most. Gradually push the stretches a little further and hold them for longer than you did in the warm-up.

Training basics

What are the building blocks of a training programme and how do they all fit together? By combining these blocks (overload, progressive overload, intensity, duration, frequency, recovery) in different ways for different sports you can stimulate a specific training effect (physical and mental) that is relevant to your sport. So, in addition to the specific skills you require for your sport, your aim is to:

- improve your body's ability to supply energy to the muscles
- strengthen and adapt the muscles involved in your sport
- develop a more efficient performance.

First, let's look at some terms you need to know and understand:

Overload
The secret of developing and improving fitness is to stress your body beyond a level normally encountered in daily activity. That is, you must 'overload' it. For example, if you exercise at a heart rate that is higher than usual, your body will adapt by becoming more efficient at that heart rate (so that sufficient oxygen is delivered for the activity).

Or, if you lift a weight that is heavier than you usually lift, your body will build up more of the correct muscle fibres to allow you to lift the weight more easily.

Progressive overload

Progression is the key, no matter how little or how low an intensity you start at. Once the body adapts to the stimulus of one particular over-load and learns to complete that movement or task more efficiently, it will then settle down again. Therefore, the degree of overload you apply (how hard you run, how much you lift) needs to be slowly and progressively increased to stop the body from becoming lazy.

Intensity

This refers to the pace (speed) at which you do any activity, or the resistance used in strength training. In other words, how hard you push yourself. Low-intensity activity implies an easy or comfortable pace, while high intensity implies a strenuous or more demanding pace requiring a greater effort. Many sports have both high- and low-intensity components, so consider both in your training programme.

Flexibility

Flexibility refers to the amount or range of movement that you have around a joint. In most normal daily activities, as well as all competi-tive and recreational sports, flexibility is important. You don't need to be as flexible as a gymnast, but improving your own range of motion by including specific stretching exercises in your training programme will help you. If these are done properly, you will notice that certain movements are easier and there is less stiffness in certain joints, par-ticularly in the morning or during extreme movements like a high reach. Good flexibility and thorough stretching also help to prevent injury. After a training session you are far more likely to pull a stiff muscle that is in a knot rather than one that has been stretched out after training. Flexibility is covered in much more detail in Chapter 6.

If the weather is fairly cool, or if you are outdoors, put on some extra clothes before you begin your cool-down.

Duration

This could be the distance or length of time taken for your whole train-ing session or the length of time taken for each repetition. Your training session usually involves alternating between intensity and duration.

Exercise does not have to be strenuous or of high intensity to have an effect. Do not be tempted to go at a faster pace than necessary: harder is not always better. To get the most out of yourself some sessions need to be hard, but the main training effect actually takes place in between the hard sessions during the rest periods. Also, you must alternate hard and easy days of training – tired muscles need time to repair.

You can keep going with higher-intensity activities for only a limited time before fatigue sets in. Lower-intensity work can last longer. The cause of fatigue is different in either case. In high-intensity exercise you usually have to stop because the accumulated waste products cause discomfort and prevent further muscle contraction (often described as a build-up of lactic acid). In easy exercise you only really need to stop when you have used up all the energy stores in the body. As you know, the faster or harder you exercise the quicker this happens.

Frequency

This usually means how many times you exercise per week. This will depend on:

- your fitness level
- the time you have available
- the type of exercise that you do from day to day.

Note that the more demanding your exercise session, the longer you will need to recover.

Recovery

In the 'recovery period' after you stop working, the work done during exercise benefits your muscles. The majority of the 'adaptations' (changes in your body and muscles) to regular exercise occur in this recovery period. The harder the exercise session, the longer the recovery required. Recovery is also essential to allow your muscles to repair the microscopic damage incurred during strenuous activity. Recovery also refers to the rest periods between bouts within an exercise session. For example, a session may consist of 6×1-minute fast bursts with 2-minute rests after each high-intensity burst. Active recovery (keeping moving at a slower pace) is better than sitting down or standing as it keeps the blood circulating and clears away waste products.

Types of physical activity

Any physical activity and the training you do for that activity can be broken into four distinct areas. These purely physical parameters are:

- aerobic conditioning
- anaerobic conditioning
- muscular strength and endurance conditioning
- flexibility conditioning.

> You have to be fit to train at your sport effectively. You become less accurate and less co-ordinated when fatigued, most noticeably in technical and tactical sports. So the longer you delay fatigue, the better you can perform in your sport. It pays to be fit!

Aerobic and anaerobic exercise

The body can break down the food you eat with or without the help of oxygen. Energy produced with oxygen is known as 'aerobic' and, in movement terms, 'aerobic activity'. Energy produced without oxygen is known as 'anaerobic' and, in movement terms, 'anaerobic activity'. Whether you use oxygen or not depends on the pace (intensity) of the activity you are doing.

Jogging in the park or playing tennis at a beginner's level are relatively low-intensity activities. In these activities, oxygen is readily available to help break down stored energy in the muscle or liver to produce energy for movement – you can keep active for a long continuous period of time. However, if you sprint or play tennis as fast and as hard as you can, after a while you will inevitably have to stop altogether or considerably reduce the intensity of your effort.

You cannot sprint for as long as you can jog, or play tennis very strenuously for prolonged periods, because your circulatory system cannot supply oxygen fast enough to support the intensity of your activity. Once the supply of oxygen is drastically reduced, the activity becomes anaerobic with the consequent build-up of lactic acid. As previously mentioned, this is a waste product of hard exercise, produced in the muscles, which prevents them from contracting. Hence it causes you to stop and the muscles to hurt.

Fortunately this occurs only at very high-effort (intensity) levels. At lower levels, lactic acid can be cleared by the aerobic system (the heart and lungs) which allows you to work for continuous periods. The fitter we are and the better our aerobic capacity, the more efficiently these waste products will be cleared away.

A good aerobic capacity is important for sports such as rugby, hockey, squash, football, basketball and some distance running. Some sports do not immediately appear to have a high aerobic endurance demand. But, if you are training for sport beyond the beginner level, you should first develop an aerobic base. You must have a good all-round level of basic fitness before you move on to specific sport-related training.

Aerobic activity is mirrored by a low to moderate rate of breathing and, not surprisingly, anaerobic work is marked by fast, laboured and strenuous breathing as the body attempts to supply enough oxygen to clear the ever-building levels of lactic acid.

You may hear of the term 'anaerobic threshold'. This describes the point when you switch over from working aerobically to working anaerobically. Some say this is when we change from exercising efficiently to inefficiently since beyond this threshold you will begin to accumulate more waste products. If you maintain this level, or increase the intensity, this accumulation of waste products will eventually make you unable to carry on. The fitter you are, the higher intensity of exercise or faster pace you can tolerate before reaching this threshold level. This is one of the important adaptations to regular training.

Muscular strength and endurance
The musculo-skeletal system (the muscles and bones) is the structure from which all movement occurs. Movement requires effort, and effort can be measured from zero (no effort), as in rest or sleep, through to 100% effort, the maximum ability at which you can run, swim, cycle, jump and so on.

Energy systems

Every movement places some demand on what is known as the 'energy systems'. These systems supply all the energy for movement by using the food you eat and the air you breathe to create the fuel which makes your muscles contract, enabling you to move. The energy for this comes from three different sources:

1. An immediate system.
2. A short-term system.
3. A long-term system.

Immediate system (anaerobic)
The ATP-CP (adenosine triphosphate-creatin phosphate) system, otherwise known as the 'alactacid' system, provides the energy for short

bursts of activity of under 10-15 seconds. Getting out of your chair, sprinting to the ball or sprinting up to 40-60 m all use this source of energy.

Short-term system (anaerobic)
This 'lactacid' system provides the energy for high-intensity activity for only 30-60 seconds, such as an intense rally in squash or a hard running period in a team game. As the name suggests, lactic acid is produced.

Long-term system (aerobic)
This system provides energy for low levels of activity almost indefinitely, as seen in marathon and ultra-marathon runners. It is also important as the base upon which the two anaerobic systems can most successfully be developed. Normal by-products are water in your breath and carbon dioxide in the air you breathe out.

But few activities use just one of these energy sources. Usually at least two, and often three, systems are used at various points in any exercise. The illustration opposite indicates how much each energy system is involved during exercise, depending on your effort. The table shows the main energy systems in a variety of sports.

Types of training

There are three main types of training:

1. Continuous (aerobic) training.
2. Interval (aerobic or anaerobic) training.
3. Resistance (anaerobic) training.
4. Flexibility training (see Chapter 6).

Continuous training
Continuous training can be any activity done at a low to moderate intensity. You should feel you are working at between 50-60% of your maximum. It should be continuous and use a large number of muscles.

Try running, swimming, cycling, rowing, stepping or circuit training. You need to train for 20-60+ minutes per session depending on your fitness. The best way to develop aerobic endurance is through running. Running is integral to most sports. Running is a whole-body, weight-bearing exercise which uses most of the body's major muscle groups. Weight-bearing activities put more impact on the joints, which is good for improving bone density, but done to excess, especially if you are overweight, can potentially contribute to joint problems.

8

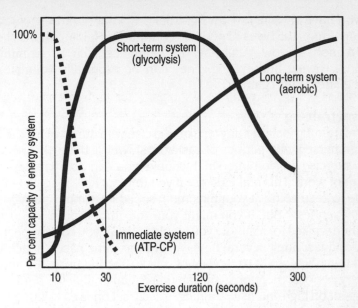

The involvement of each energy system during different durations of exercise

Major systems	Performance time	Examples of physical activities
ATP-CP	less than 20 seconds	shot-put, 100-m sprint, base stealing, golf and tennis swings
ATP-CP and anaerobic glycolysis (lactic acid)	from about 30 seconds to 90 seconds	200-m to 400-m sprints, speed skating, 100-m swim
anaerobic glycolysis (lactic acid) and aerobic	from about 90 seconds to several minutes	800-m dash, gymnastics events, boxing (3 min rounds), wrestling (2 min periods)
aerobic	more than several minutes	football and lacrosse (except goalies), cross-country skiing, marathon run, jogging

The main energy systems used in different sports

If you have an injury to a weight-bearing joint or muscle (such as the hamstring), the types of aerobic/continuous training that will suit you are non- or low-weight-bearing activities such as swimming, stepping, rowing and cycling. They can be especially valuable for training after a hard game.

Interval training

Interval training includes any type of exercise with bursts of hard activity interspersed with periods of easier or slower activity. By breaking up an exercise session into small chunks you can do a greater total amount of work. This makes sense if you think of how long you might be able to keep going at your maximum speed – a minute, perhaps, or maybe even less? But, if you ran at your maximum speed for 20 seconds then walked for a minute you would find that you could repeat the 20-second fast burst several times and at the same pace. In fact, you would be able to do 6-10 repeats of this 20-second burst. By adding recovery periods, therefore, you can more than double the amount of time spent on high-intensity training: 9×20 seconds equalling 3 minutes, compared to only 1 minute if continuous.

The way your training is put together depends on the effect you are aiming for. Generally, you use longer duration and less intense intervals with a short recovery time to improve aerobic capacity. This may be something like 8×2 minutes steady pace running with 1 minute recovery, or $12\text{-}15 \times 200$ m stride-outs with 30-60 seconds recovery.

Pace yourself. Intervals are not always flat-out bursts. If you start the first few too fast, you won't be able to finish such a session.

At the other end of the interval training spectrum are fast-pace workbouts where you are aiming for close to maximum speed during the intervals, with a much longer recovery period. To maintain the quality of the intervals you need a full recovery. For example, sets of running 4×50 m with a walk-back recovery after each 50 m and 5-minute rests between sets. These are the two extremes – you choose the variation that best suits your needs. All you do is adjust the speed, duration and recovery.

Resistance training

Resistance training is dealt with fully in Chapter 5, so this is just a brief overview. The term 'resistance training' applies to the muscular system and includes any form of training that puts an overload on the muscles. This causes them to get stronger, develop better endurance, and become bigger or more explosive and powerful. The methods commonly used to provide resistance training are:

- manual resistance, whereby your own body weight or that of a partner would provide the resistance. Example: a press-up
- isometric resistance, whereby you contract a muscle(s) against an immovable object. Example: holding a weight at arm's length
- elastic resistance methods using elastic tubes and bands
- resistance running on hills and in water and other devices which cause resistance
- the use of weights. This is by far the most effective and widespread method of resistance training. Weight training is a convenient, variable and low-cost way of improving muscular strength. Through a variety of repetitions (the number of times you perform a given exercise), sets (the number of given repetitions) and the type of exercise you perform you can ensure improvement will take place. The majority of weight-training machines are very safe and effective but always make sure that you receive qualified advice when resistance training (in fact, any sort of training), especially if it is to encompass free weights such as dumbbells and barbells.

CHAPTER 2

Self Assessment
(Are You Ready?)

Even if you already take regular exercise, it's important to review your general level of health and fitness from time to time. This helps you to find out if there is anything wrong before you start exercising, and also allows you to monitor your fitness and measure your progress. In this chapter you'll find health and lifestyle questionnaires and some basic fitness tests to help you assess your current 'readiness for exercise'. You will also find out how to measure your body mass index (BMI) and hip-to-waist ratio; how to test specific areas such as your stomach muscles and upper-body strength; and how to use the results as a base line from which to record the improvements you make. The advanced self-assessment tests starting on page 24 should be attempted only by people who already take regular exercise, or after you have reached the goals set out in the beginner's training programmes for any particular sport in this book.

FIRST THINGS FIRST

If you are a beginner, or returning to sport after a long break, start your self assessment by answering these simple questions about your state of health and follow the advice given afterwards.

General health questionnaire

- Have you ever had pains in your head or chest?   Yes ☐ No ☐

- Do you often feel faint or have spells of severe dizziness?   Yes ☐ No ☐

- Has your doctor ever told you that you have high blood pressure?   Yes ☐ No ☐

- Has your doctor ever told you that you have a bone or joint problem that might be made worse by exercise?   Yes ☐ No ☐

- Has your doctor ever told you that you have heart trouble?   Yes ☐ No ☐

- Have any of your close relatives suffered from any heart-related condition (e.g. angina, coronary heart disease, stroke or heart surgery)?   Yes ☐ No ☐

- Is there any good physical reason that has not been mentioned here why you should not follow an exercise programme?   Yes ☐ No ☐

Any yes answers?
You should consult your doctor before going any further with the self assessment or exercise programmes. Check that it is safe for you to go ahead.

All no answers?
Go on to the next stage of self assessment or, if you prefer, get straight on with your chosen exercise programme.

If you have been ill enough to be off work or in bed for one day or more in the past two weeks, postpone your exercise plans for a week. If you continue to feel below par, consult your doctor.

13

Lifestyle awareness questionnaire

Now it's time to answer – truthfully – some questions about your lifestyle. Nobody else is going to see your answers, so there's no point in fooling yourself about how healthily you live.

1. Are you a non-smoker? ☐ Yes ☐ No
   If no, how many do you smoke per day?

   cigarettes: ☐ 40 or more ☐ 20-39

   ☐ 10-19 ☐ 1-9

   cigars/pipes: ☐ 5 or more, or any inhaled

   ☐ less than 5, none inhaled

2. Do you take steps to control or reduce stress in
   your life? For example, do you take time to sit
   and relax, get enough sleep, do breathing
   exercises, meditate? ☐ Yes ☐ No

3. If you drink alcohol, do you:
   a) Drink fewer than 14 (for women) or
      21 (for men) units per week? ☐ Yes ☐ No
   b) Drink fewer than 3 (for women) or
      5 (for men) units on any single day? ☐ Yes ☐ No

4. Do you usually spend at least 20 minutes
   exercising most days of the week? ☐ Yes ☐ No

5. Do you think you are the correct weight
   for your frame size and height? ☐ Yes ☐ No

6. Can you walk 4 miles briskly without
   getting tired? ☐ Yes ☐ No

7. Do you have your blood pressure measured
   once a year? ☐ Yes ☐ No

8. Do you do the following things regarding your diet:
   a) Avoid eating too many high-fat foods and
      foods containing cholesterol? ☐ Yes ☐ No
   b) Avoid eating too much sugar and sweet
      foods? ☐ Yes ☐ No
   c) Include plenty of fibre and fresh food in
      your diet, e.g. cereals, fruits and vegetables? ☐ Yes ☐ No

Any no answers?

If you answered no to any of the questions, you should be aware of the following points in relation to each question:

1. If you are still smoking, starting to exercise regularly will probably help you want to stop, or at least cut down.
2. If you feel stressed, try some of the suggestions given. To find out more about what causes stress and how to control it, see the books suggested in the bibliography or consult your GP.
3. Drinking more than the limits of alcohol given may affect your general health and will adversely affect your sporting performance. On average, try to stay within the recommended limits.
4. Ideally, you should try to take some light exercise most days – at least some brisk walking. Taking some moderately intense exercise three or four times a week is a good average.
5. If you are overweight, starting to exercise will help you to trim down, especially if you also pay attention to your diet.
6. If a brisk 4-mile walk tires you, you should start training only gently. Or, if this is due to a medical condition, consult your doctor.
7. Your GP will measure your blood pressure for you. It's a good idea to have it checked once a year as part of a general check-up.
8. If you don't already follow these diet suggestions, try to become more aware of what you can do to improve your diet (see the books in the bibliography and Chapter 11).

Basic fitness tests

Next, here are some exercises to test your present fitness level. Repeat the same tests every 6-8 weeks as you follow your exercise programme to measure your progress. To make sure you get accurate results, try to keep test conditions consistent, and check them by noting the following each time you test yourself:

- the time of day
- whether you exercised or did anything strenuous the same day or the day before
- the weather: is it warm, cold, wet or dry (outside)?
- that you didn't drink coffee or smoke just before the test.

It's much more fun to do these tests with other people. You may get better results, too. You push yourself just a little harder if a friend is competing with you or timing you.

Aerobic fitness, or stamina (staying power), is a good way to tell how fit you are generally. Try either of the following stamina tests, then work out your stamina level using the maximum aerobic capacity (VO$_2$ max) equation as explained on pages 18–19.

The Cooper 12-minute walk/run test*

This test, named after top American physiologist Dr Kenneth Cooper, tests your fitness based on the distance you can cover in exactly 12 minutes. You can walk or run the test, depending on how fit you are. It is what is called a 'maximal test', which means you should make your very best effort, so run if you can.

1. Before you start, do a light warm-up (see Chapter 1).
2. Mark your starting point. This is easy on a standard, all-weather running track which has a start line. If you do the test on the street, mark the start with chalk or any object that will stay in place.
3. Start walking or running when you are ready. Start a stopwatch, or note the exact time by the second hand of a wristwatch. Go at your best speed, allowing for the fact that you must keep it up for 12 minutes.
4. Stop walking or running after exactly 12 minutes (this is where it helps if a friend can keep an eye on the time). Mark your stopping point.
5. Measure how far you have walked or run. Again, this is easy to do on a track, where every lap is 400 m. If you did the test on the street, use your car's milometer to measure the distance. Use this distance to calculate your maximum aerobic capacity in the equation on page 19 or in the interpretation table shown opposite.

The 1½-mile run test*

This is an alternative way to test your stamina. You may find this test easier to set up.

1. Measure out a 1½-mile distance as accurately as you can (use a running track or milometer, as described before).
2. After a gentle warm-up (see Chapter 1), try to cover the 1½ miles in the fastest possible time. Record the time in minutes and seconds.
3. Now use this time to calculate your maximum aerobic capacity by consulting the following interpretation table:

*From R. Hockey, *Physical Fitness: The Pathway to Healthful Living* (1993) 7th edition. Reproduced with permission of the McGraw-Hill Companies.

Estimated maximal VO$_2$ based on 12-minute run and 1½-mile run tests

1½-mile run time (min:sec)	12-minute run distance (miles)	estimated maximal VO$_2$ (ml/kg body weight/min)
8:42	2.07	56
8:54	2.02	55
9:03	1.99	54
9:17	1.94	53
9:25	1.91	52
9:38	1.87	51
9:50	1.83	50
10:03	1.79	49
10.17	1.75	48
10:32	1.71	47
10:50	1.66	46
11:06	1.62	45
11:24	1.58	44
11:41	1.54	43
12:00	1.50	42
12:25	1.45	41
12:46	1.41	40
13:08	1.37	39
13:32	1.33	38
13:57	1.29	37
14:31	1.24	36
15:00	1.20	35
15:31	1.16	34
16:04	1.12	33
16:40	1.08	32
17:28	1.03	31
18:10	0.99	30
18:57	0.95	29
19:46	0.91	28
20:41	0.87	27
21:41	0.83	26
23:05	0.78	25

Maximum aerobic capacity: interpretation table, from R. Hockey, Physical Fitness: The Pathway to Healthful Living *(1993) 7th edition. Reproduced with permission of The McGraw-Hill Companies.*

The shuttle run test

This is a stamina test you may come across if you train with a club, particularly a hockey or football club. The test involves running backwards and forwards between a starting point and markers at a set distance (20 m) apart. At the same time you play a special cassette. Timed beeps on the tape gradually allow you less and less time to make the runs. When you can no longer reach the markers within the time limits, the level you managed to reach is used in calculating your VO_2 max. It's a very good test, and the cassette is available from the National Coaching Foundation, 114 Cardigan Road, Headingley, Leeds LS6 3BJ, telephone number 0113 274 4802.

Maximum aerobic capacity

Calculating your maximum aerobic capacity (or VO_2 max) is a good indicator of your stamina. It calculates the maximum amount of oxygen that you can take in through your lungs for your muscles to use during exercise. The higher the figure, the fitter you are. Here's

Maximal oxygen consumption (ml/kg/min)

Age	Below average		Average
	Very poor	Poor	Fair
Women			
18–29	below 30.6	30.6–33.7	33.8–36.6
30–39	below 28.7	28.7–32.2	32.3–34.5
40–49	below 26.5	26.5–29.4	29.5–32.2
50–59	below 24.3	24.3–26.8	26.9–29.3
60 and over	below 22.8	22.8–24.4	24.5–27.1
Men			
18–29	below 37.1	37.1–40.9	41.0–44.1
30–39	below 35.4	35.4–38.8	38.9–42.3
40–49	below 33.0	33.0–36.7	36.8–39.8
50–59	below 30.2	30.2–33.7	33.8–36.6
60 and over	below 26.5	26.5–30.1	30.2–33.5

Source: based on norms from *The Physical Fitness Specialist Manual*, The Cooper Institute for Aerobics Research, Dallas, Texas; used with permission.

how to work out your VO_2 max from the Cooper 12-minute walk/run test:

$$(35.97 \times \text{distance in miles}) - 11.29 = VO_2 \text{ max}$$

Here's an example:

If a woman covers $1\frac{1}{2}$ miles in the 12-minute test, her estimated aerobic capacity is:

$$(35.97 \times 1.5) - 11.29 = 53.96 - 11.29$$
$$= 42.67 \text{ ml/kg/min}$$

VO_2 max is expressed in millilitres (ml) of oxygen per kilogram (kg) of body weight per minute, or 'ml/kg/min'. It is expressed in relation to body weight because the available oxygen has to circulate throughout your whole body all the time you are exercising. Work out your VO_2 max and compare it with others of the same sex and age in the table below:

Above average		
Good	Excellent	Superior
36.7–40.9	41.0–46.7	above 46.7
34.6–38.5	38.6–43.8	above 43.8
32.3–36.2	36.3–40.9	above 40.9
29.4–32.2	32.3–36.7	above 36.7
27.2–31.1	31.2–37.4	above 37.4
44.2–48.1	48.2–53.9	above 53.9
42.4–46.7	46.8–52.4	above 52.4
39.9–44.0	44.1–50.3	above 50.3
36.7–40.9	41.0–47.0	above 47.0
33.6–38.0	38.1–45.1	above 45.1

Results

If your score is 'below average', you've got quite a lot of work to do, but the only way is up. 'Average' means just what it says, but it is calculated from results of a wide cross-section of people, not just sports people. You'll want to improve if you're going to enjoy your sport. 'Above average' is what you should aim for. Anyone involved in sport at a competitive level should be at the top end of this category.

Are you the right weight?

The usual height and weight tables you see give you a very rough guide to the correct weight for your height. But they don't take into account the size of your frame (whether you have big bones or not) or whether the weight is made up of a large amount of fat (generally a disadvantage) or muscle (often an advantage). The best way to find out if you are the right weight is to have a body fat test, which you can have done at a gym or fitness assessment centre. This tells you how much fat you are carrying, whether this is too much or too little, and how much you can afford to lose.

If you can't easily get tested, the next best measure is to work out your body mass index (BMI). This is a simple way to work out your weight in proportion to your height. You need to know your weight in kilograms and your height in metres.

The formula is: BMI = weight (kg) ÷ height × height

Here's an example:

If you weigh 63 kg and your height is 174 cm (1.74 m)
multiply 1.74 by 1.74 to get 3.028
Then divide 63 by 3.028 = 20.08 (your BMI)

BMI results
- a BMI of below 20 is below normal weight
- a BMI of 20-25 is ideal, with lower being better for more athletic people
- a BMI of 25-30 is overweight
- a BMI of over 30 is considered obese.

Waist-to-hip ratio

There are probably parts of your body that you would like to see changing and improving during the course of your exercise programme. Apart from being very satisfying, such changes are also a useful measure of your fitness progress. One good thing to measure is your waist-to-hip ratio.

Experts have proved that people who carry excess weight around their abdomen (middle) are less healthy and even die earlier than people who put weight on elsewhere (hips and thighs, for example). Excess fat around your major organs makes them work harder and wear out more quickly. A simple measure you can do to assess your risk is this waist:hip ratio test:

> Measure around your hips and waist with a good tape measure, in centimetres. Divide the waist measure by the hip measure to get your ratio.

Example: waist = 29 in
                hip   = 36 in
                ratio = 0.8 (29 ÷ 36)

An average guide is that you want the ratio to be under or close to 1. Ideally, a man should be under 0.95 and a woman under 0.85. Exercising will help you reduce the ratio.

Body measurements

Another good way to measure your progress is to keep a check on your body shape and size. You can do this effectively by taking these four measurements:

1. Your abdomen – around the belly button.
2. Your hips – around the widest part.
3. Your thigh – measure a specific distance up from your knee so you can measure at exactly the same spot next time.
4. Your upper arm – again, measure a distance, this time up from your elbow to the widest part of the biceps.

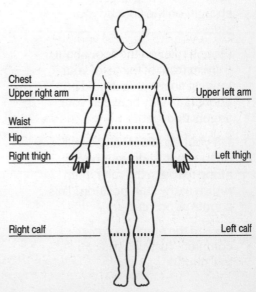

Chest
Upper right arm
Upper left arm
Waist
Hip
Right thigh
Left thigh
Right calf
Left calf

Keep a note of these measurements and try them again later to see if there have been any improvements. Don't re-do them until you've done at least 2 months of regular training – you'll only be disappointed. The best time to do it is when you repeat all the tests in this section as a complete reassessment.

Targeted tests

The next 2 tests are for specific parts of your body that are important in most sports and can affect overall performance.

The tummy crunch or sit-up

Although the stomach (abdomen) may not seem directly relevant to many sports, the tummy muscles play an extremely important supporting role in any activity, and help posture, too, which is important. Weak or out-of-condition abdominal muscles can cause poor posture, sometimes leading to back pain, and leaving you more susceptible to back injuries. Abdominal strength and endurance is one aspect of fitness that you can develop as part of your training programme and which could help you avoid injury, so it's well worth testing.

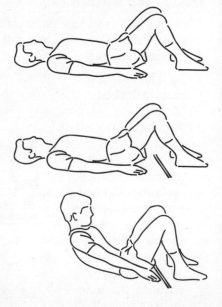

1. Lie on your back on the floor, with your knees bent and hip-width apart. Have your hands palms down and fingers straight on the floor by your sides.

2. Place a ruler on the floor about 8 cm in front of the tip of your longest finger (this should be about half-way between your fingers and feet).

3. Lift your shoulders and chest off the floor, slide your hands along to touch the ruler, then return to the start position. This counts as one curl-up.

4. Record the number of complete curl-ups you can do in 1 minute.

Ask a friend to watch and make sure you do sit-ups and press-ups correctly. No cheating allowed!

Classic press-ups

Press-ups give a good indication of your upper-body strength and endurance, particularly of the muscles in your chest, shoulders and the back of the arm (triceps). Even in sports where legs seem to do the majority of the work, the upper body and arms are important. Good upper-body strength and arm movement can help you move your whole body more efficiently.

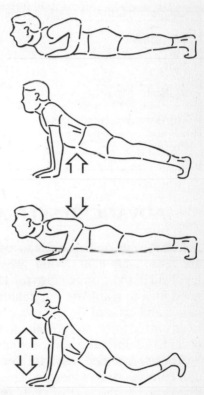

1. Lie on the floor on your stomach with your hands on the floor beside your shoulders.
2. From here, push your body up to straighten your arms. Keep your back straight.
3. Lower your body by bending at the elbows to about 15 cm from the floor. This is one complete press-up.
4. Record the number of complete press-ups you do in 1 minute.

Press-ups tip: if you cannot manage a full press-up, modify the exercise by keeping your knees rather than your feet on the floor, then do the exercise in the same way.

KEEP A RECORD

Do all the tests in this chapter every 2-3 months as you follow your training programme. If you wish, you can keep the results in the form of a table like the one shown on page 24. You'll probably be encouraged as you see quite large changes to start with. Don't be put off if improvements then begin to slow down. This is quite normal. In fact, improvements continue but your body will be adapting in other ways that these tests can't measure.

Record table for self-assessment results

Date: _____ _____ _____

Weight: _____ _____ _____

Cooper distance/ 1 ½ -mile time: _____ _____ _____

VO$_2$ max: _____ _____ _____

BMI: _____ _____ _____

Waist-to-hip ratio: _____ _____ _____

Tummy crunch/sit-up score: _____ _____ _____

Press-up score: _____ _____ _____

ADVANCED SELF-ASSESSMENT TESTS

Before moving on to the advanced tests below it is important that you are reasonably fit (in other words, you should have been actively involved in sport or exercise for 12 weeks or more). In any case, it's a good idea to complete the health and lifestyle awareness questionnaires and general fitness tests earlier in this chapter before going on to advanced tests, as you will often need to know basic fitness data in order to interpret the advanced test results.

These advanced tests are known as 'performance tests' as they don't just measure aspects of fitness in isolation, but assess activities that relate to the sort of skills you use in an actual game. For this reason, they give you a good idea of how effective your training has been. The results of these tests may be a little less precise than those of more basic tests, depending on how carefully you set them up, but they are well worth doing, as they cost nothing, are reliable enough to show improvement or a drop in performance, and are relatively quick and easy to perform.

Test conditions

As in the basic tests, make sure the results are as accurate as possible by performing all the tests under similar conditions. These guidelines will help you:

1. Always use the same test. There are several different tests to measure any one thing.
2. Ensure external conditions are the same – whether you are indoors or outdoors, the weather, what you wear and so on.
3. Drink plenty of liquids such as water, sports drinks, etc.
4. Do not:
   - eat less than 1 hour before testing
   - take caffeine (coffee, Coca-Cola, etc.), smoke or drink alcohol less than 3-4 hours before testing
   - test if you are feeling unwell or have just recovered from an illness or injury.

Strength-assessment test

Strength is the most difficult aspect of fitness to assess, as pure strength is defined as the maximum you can lift in just 1 attempt. Anything more than 1 attempt technically becomes muscle endurance. However, it always takes more than 1 attempt to achieve your maximum lifting weight (a warm-up and a few trial lifts), which means that purists would say it doesn't record a true maximum. However, getting as close as you can to a one-repetition maximum lift is still a reasonable way to assess performance strength. Most experts agree that 3, 5 or 10 attempts – called a 3, 5 or 10 repetition maximum (RM) – are acceptable. Just remember that the result will also include a muscle endurance element and, obviously, you should use the same number of lifts each time you test.

How to do a 3, 5 or 10 RM lift
Before you do this test, make sure you are fully warmed up and have no injuries. It is vital to have at least 1 assistant, or spotter, who can 'catch' the weight when you become exhausted. (You may wish to use the Self Assessment scoring sheet on page 27.)

1. Choose which lifting exercise you will use to determine your maximum lift. For example, a bench press is popular, or you could try a leg press or shoulder press. Whichever exercise you choose, make sure you know how to do it correctly. If you're not sure, ask a trained member of staff at the gym.

2. Select a weight you feel is near your maximum. This is not easy to judge the first time you do the test. Make your best guess and adjust as suggested below.

3. Attempt to lift the weight the number of times (repetitions) you have chosen (3, 5 or 10). Your spotter(s) must be on watch all the time and be ready to assist at any point.

4. Record the weight you succeeded in lifting the number of times you were attempting.

5. If you find your first attempt too easy, rest for at least 5 minutes before trying a new weight. Use a smaller weight if your first estimate was too high.

> Remember – you are trying to lift your maximum, not just above or below it.

The table opposite shows you how to record your score. You need to look out for how your maximum weights increase, decrease or remain constant.

Assessing power test

Power (P) is defined as the maximum force you can exert in the shortest time. It is expressed in an equation, like this:

$$P = \text{force} \times \text{distance}$$

Power is normally measured by various forms of bounds and jumps. The following jump and reach exercise is a standard measure of power and, providing you jump using the same technique in each test, you can expect to get a realistic measure of change.

For this test you need:

- a wall
- a good, flat, solid surface to jump off
- a graduated measure or some chalk.

1. Stand side-on to the wall (by the measure if you have one). Reach up with the arm next to the wall, hand extended and fingers pointing up. Keep your feet flat on the floor, use a natural (not over-stretched) reach and note where your longest finger stretches to on the marker. Ask a friend to record this height. If you don't have a marker, rub coloured chalk on your fingertip before making your reach and mark the wall, then measure the height.

Self Assessment scoring sheet

Name: _____ Date: _____

Age: _____   Position: _____   Height: _____   Weight: _____

Cooper 12-minute run score: | laps: _____ metres: _____ score: _____ |

Queens College step test score: _____

Body composition: Body mass index: _____

Waist:hip ratio: _____

Circumferences:

Chest: _____

Waist: _____

Hip: _____

Upper arm: _____

Thigh: _____

Calf: _____

Repeated maximum lifts (RM) for strength assessment

Exercise	3 RM (kg)	5 RM (kg)	10 RM (kg)
Bench press			
Leg press			
Shoulder press			

One-minute press-up score: _____

One-minute sit-up score: _____

15 m score: | T1: ___ T2: ___ T3: ___ | Best: ___ |

30 m score: | T1: ___ T2: ___ T3: ___ | Best: ___ |

Jump & reach score: | T1: ___ T2: ___ T3: ___ | Best: ___ |

Repeated shuttle score:

trial 1 __   trial 2 __   trial 3 __   trial 4 __   trial 5 __   trial 6 __

Max score: _____   Min score: _____   Fatigue factor: _____

Notes:

2. From a normal standing position, hands by your side, jump and reach up to touch the wall as high as you can (again, get your helper to observe the marker or use chalk on your fingertip. You could also stick a sheet of blank paper on the wall and colour the top of your finger with a felt-tip pen).
3. Don't step into the jump but do it from both feet on the ground. Swing your arms if you like, and bend your knees to spring, but try to keep these elements as consistent as possible for each jump. Your partner should record the distance between your first and second mark.

Acceleration and speed test

Acceleration is defined as the rate of increase in velocity – velocity being the rate at which an object (in this case you) travels in a given direction. Speed is the maximum rate of velocity. Knowing how fast you are (speed) and how quickly you can 'get off the mark' (acceleration) is the key to many sporting activities. Most people think speed is the most crucial aspect of any sport in which moving (usually, running) is important. But if you look closely at most team or racquet sports, you'll see that very little pure speed is involved. If a player needs to run in one direction for 30 m or so, pure speed is handy. But in most sports, players run in a variety of directions (side-stepping, etc.), or for less than 15 m before they change directions, often slowing down and speeding up to do so. In this case, acceleration (how quickly they can get to top speed from a halt) is obviously the main requirement.

To assess acceleration and speed you need to do 2 short runs:

1. A 15-m sprint, allowing you to just reach top speed.
2. A 30-m sprint to assess pure speed.

To perform these tests you need:

- a flat, even running surface. It should have good grip and be consistent. A gym floor or running track is ideal.
- a stopwatch and a floor tape to mark the distances.

1. Stand with the toe of your leading foot just behind the start mark. Ask a helper to stand in line with the finish mark so that he can see when you cross the line.
2. Start running whenever you like. The helper starts the stopwatch as soon as he sees movement.
3. The instant you cross the finish mark the helper stops the watch.

4. Do this for both 15 m and 30 m distances. Run each distance 3 times and record the best time for each. You need to be fully recovered from each attempt before trying again.

Speed endurance test

As explained on pages 15–19, there are several tests you can use to calculate aerobic capacity. This is fundamental to sporting activity at all levels, so even fitter people should take one of these tests first. The overall 'pace' at which any sport or game is played relies directly on your aerobic capacity. At more advanced levels, players work at the very limits of this capacity. This means they are drawing on both speed and endurance, so the person who can play consistently at the highest possible rate without tiring will often perform best. Measuring speed endurance, along with general aerobic capacity, therefore becomes important at advanced levels.

You test speed endurance by alternating 'work bouts' with 'rest bouts'. The aim of this test is for the runner to cover as much distance as possible each time and to keep that distance consistent over 6 repetitions.

To perform this test you will need:

- a flat, non-slip surface such as a track or gymnasium. You can do it on grass, but it should not be wet or uneven
- a stopwatch or wristwatch with a second hand
- a tape measure to mark 5-m intervals for a total distance of 20 m from the start point.

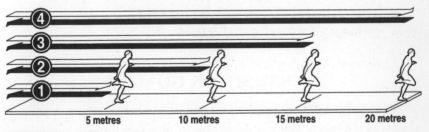

| 5 metres | 10 metres | 15 metres | 20 metres |

Speed endurance test marked at 5-m intervals

1. Begin with the toe of your leading foot just behind the start mark.
2. The recorder yells 'Go' and simultaneously starts the stopwatch.
3. You sprint to the 1st mark, place a foot on it and return to the start, then run to the 2nd mark and back to the start, and so on to the 3rd and 4th marks and back.

4. Continue until the recorder shouts 'Rest' after exactly 30 seconds. If you complete the run to the 4th marker and back before time is up, start again by running to the 1st marker and back, and so on.
5. Stop at the rest signal. Return to the start mark if you are not there already. The recorder times 35 seconds of rest.
6. After 35 seconds, the recorder shouts 'Go' once more, and you start again, repeating the whole exercise.
7. Repeat the exercise 4 more times (shuttle run 6 times altogether).

Scoring

The exact point you reach at the end of each 30-second running bout should be recorded to the nearest 5 m (each time you run between markers it's 5 m both there and back).

For example:

- If you complete 1 full shuttle (out and back to all 4 markers), that's 100 m.
- If you continue to run and reach the 2nd mark again, that's another 20 m.
- If you stop between 2 markers and are close to half-way between, you are credited with the 5 m.
- You are not credited if you have only just completed a turn.

Note the difference between the highest distance you covered and the lowest distance over the 6 attempts. This is called the 'fatigue factor'.

Fatigue factor = maximum distance − minimum distance

You should try to reduce your fatigue factor, achieving a more consistent, and longer, distance over all 6 runs.

TRANSITION GOALS

Each sport or group of sports in this book is approached first from a beginner's (entry-level) point of view. At the end of each beginner's section you will find some 'transition goals'. These are intended as an easy guide to determine whether you are ready to move on to (or, even, begin at) the advanced level. The transition goals are tailored to specific sports and it is essential that you meet all the goals to ensure that you move on safely and sensibly. Some transition goals are common to many sports, but don't assume that being ready for advanced training in one sport is enough to allow advanced training in another.

Transition goals cover such things as:

- physical goals, such as aerobic capacity, strength, muscle endurance, flexibility
- equipment: do you need to upgrade?
- training habits: diet, frequency of training and so on.

In general, transition goals require you to complete a certain percentage of a suggested programme within a certain time. This ensures you have the base you need to move safely to the advanced level.

Other tests

As well as transition goals, in each section you will find general fitness assessment and, if appropriate, advanced fitness assessment tests. These are not obligatory, but purely for your own interest.

CHAPTER 3

Periodization
(Your Training Year)

Even if you managed to avoid boredom, it would be difficult to reach your long-term fitness, strength and performance goals by doing the same training programme week after week, or month after month. Your physical gains would slow down and there would be an increased risk of overuse injuries or imbalances in muscles that were being repeatedly used in the same way.

For this reason the training year (or indeed any time period) is broken up into planned blocks or cycles, each working towards specific targets. This approach applies whether you are exercising for weight loss and health benefits or whether you are training regularly for a particular sport. The whole training process is about getting the timing right through manipulation of the basic training tools – volume, intensity, duration – and the body's adaptation to these stresses by maintaining everything in a state of balance.

PREPARING FOR SPORT

Professional trainers tend to plan training on a yearly basis. For any sport there will be an element of physical, technical and tactical preparation. Each needs emphasizing in different degrees in training at different times in the year.

Break down your sport into the different stages of preparation. If you are a beginner, just taking up or getting back into a sport, this may be a little more difficult as you may not be so concerned about reaching your peak or optimal fitness level for any particular competitive season. However, at the end of a year you may find yourself going through the transition stages outlined later in this book, and considering taking up the sport more competitively. Even if this just entails joining a local club to play once every week or every other week, you should still find that there are definite peak phases in the year when more people take part and the competition is tougher. You can consider these the times when you want to be playing or performing at your best.

If you are already involved in a sport, not necessarily at a serious level, you will find that there are definite competitive seasons at set times of the year. For example, cyclists and triathletes typically race from April to October; footballers, rugby and hockey and basketball players compete from September to April. In running you can race at any time of the year, although there is a definite winter cross-country season. Therefore, your competitive season is the race or races that you have decided to aim for – a 10-km race perhaps or even a marathon – and you can work backwards from there.

We tend, therefore, to break the training year down into basic areas of preparation, each of which can be further broken down:

- preparation
- competition
- transition or recovery.

First identify your competitive season, or when you want to reach your peak and then work backwards from there.

STAGES OF TRAINING

Preparation: 1st stage – lasts 4-12 weeks

This is a very important stage and should not be rushed. The aim is to develop all-round fitness and general conditioning. The training in this stage is at a low intensity and the volume or amount will progress from low to moderate. The progression involves a gradual increase in duration, working on increasing your endurance and development of a sound basis of aerobic fitness. This stage *prepares* you for the later training stages.

Preparation: 2nd stage – lasts 4-12 weeks

Here the focus is on progressively increasing the duration and then the intensity or pace. This is the hard-work stage and the emphasis is on quality rather than the quantity of the 1st stage. At the end of this stage you should be approaching a good and consistent level of fitness.

Competition: 1st stage – 8-12 weeks

This 1st stage utilizes your already well-developed overall fitness resulting from your hard work in the first 2 preparation stages where you developed sports-specific fitness and skills. In this stage the intensity increases while the volume of training decreases. A lot more time is here dedicated towards skill and tactical training. At the end of this stage you should feel at your best, in terms of fitness and skill.

Competition: 2nd stage – 4-12+ weeks

Now is the time of year when your sport has most of its competition or you have most of your matches, games or races. This is when you want to be feeling at your physical best, fitness- and skill-wise. The hard work has been done by this stage and now you want to feel the benefits. Training volume is much lower in this stage as you focus on maintaining fitness and doing higher-intensity workouts to 'sharpen' your fitness. The volume also decreases because you need to reduce your training, or rest just before each game, match or race. You have more days off in this stage. For example, if you are playing a football or rugby match every Saturday, you will need to have an easy day of training, or the whole day off, on Friday, play on Saturday, and have an easy training recovery day on Sunday. The length of this stage varies according to your sport and the length of the competition season.

Transition or recovery stage – 4 weeks or longer

After all these stages the transition or recovery stage is well earned. Now is when you give yourself to recovery, both physically and psychologically. An active approach in this stage is best to keep your fitness 'ticking over': do any activities that you enjoy. This gives your muscles a respite while allowing you to maintain your fitness.

Then the whole cycle can repeat itself as you go back into the preparation phase for the next year or season.

Single periodized year											
months	Nov	Dec	Jan	Feb	Mar	Apr	May	Jun	Jul	Aug	Sep	Oct
phases	1				2		3		4		5	6
periods	preparation						competition					transition

> Keep a training record or log so you can look back at what you did in previous years, compare performances and see what worked or did not work. (See Appendix 1 for examples of record sheets.)

Planning

As well as these long-term patterns of training, taking in weeks at a time, each week in itself forms its own cycle or pattern. You may train with a club on certain days or evenings, or run longer runs on a Saturday or Sunday. Here are some important things to consider:

- Plan your week in advance to see when and where you can fit in your training. This will depend on your lifestyle and the demands of a particular week.
- The plan must be flexible. You should be able to adapt it if commitments change, whether work or travel or family.

It is much easier and less stressful to train beneficially if you are following a realistic (particularly in terms of time) progression. When you are training you should be able to focus on just that. Also, make friends and family aware of your training times.

CHAPTER 4

Aerobic Training
(Training Heart Rate)

Training for any sport or event is not just a matter of going out and running, cycling, swimming or whatever as fast as possible until you collapse in a heap, exhausted. Each type of training session is designed to work on different areas and to achieve differing but complementary physical results. Slow- and easy-pace training has just as important a role to play as those demanding, high-intensity interval training sessions. It is important to realize that all training does not have to be strenuous or exhausting to be effective.

THE HEART RATE

Throughout this book, and particularly in the individual sports sections, different types of session will be described in terms of a particular pace, recovery time or heart rate. The easiest way to monitor the pace or intensity of a workout is by using the heart rate.

The heart rate reflects the demands placed on the cardiovascular system – the heart, lungs and blood vessels – at any time. The heart is responsible for pumping the oxygen-rich blood to the muscles. The muscles use the oxygen to release energy from their energy stores. The harder we push ourselves, the faster the heart has to beat. Measuring the heart can be used to:

- control the pace of a workout
- see how quickly you recover
- gauge how hard you are working.

However, you must listen to other physical messages or cues in order to monitor the demand or stress of a session. These may include breathing rate, muscle fatigue or soreness, co-ordination and balance, all of which affect how you cope with a session.

Resting heart rate

The resting heart rate also shows if we are a bit 'under the weather', generally tired or coming down with an illness, such as a cold. At times like this the resting heart rate may be about 5-10 beats higher than normal for a few days. Take your resting heart rate first thing in the morning or after you have been sitting or lying for at least half an hour. Get to know your resting heart rate. Once you are confident in taking the measurement, record it every morning for a week and keep a record, perhaps in your training diary. The next time you are feeling run down or tired, measure your resting heart rate in the same way and at the same time of day and compare it to this record. If it is 10 beats higher than this, it is time to rest or take it easy for the day and perhaps to skip your training on that day. Regular training causes a drop in your resting heart rate over time.

Measuring heart rate manually

There are two major arteries that are easy to locate and that are usually used for pulse counts. These are (1) the *carotid* artery in the neck just to the left or right of the windpipe and (2) the *radial* pulse at the wrist just above the base of the thumb.

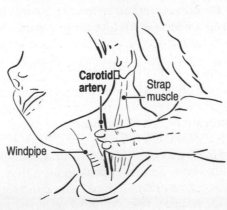

Where to find the carotid artery

- Always use the fingertips (index and middle finger) rather than the thumb to take a measurement, as the thumb has a pulse itself. Move the fingers until you find a strong pulse and press gently so as not to disrupt the blood flow. The carotid pulse is probably the easier one to measure and it tends to be quite strong during or after exercise.

- Pulse rate is measured in beats per minute. You can either count the pulse for a whole minute, or count it in parts of a minute and then multiply to get beats per minute. After exercise it is better to measure for parts of a minute, as your heart rate slows very quickly when you stop exercising. The key is to locate the pulse quickly and to count the rate for a short period of time.

- Use a digital watch or a watch with a clear second hand and begin counting with 0 rather than 1 (0-1-2-3).

- Keep moving while you are locating the pulse and then stop when you are taking a count.

- Count the beats for 10 (multiply by 6) or 15 (multiply by 4) seconds and then multiply by the appropriate figure to get beats per minute.

Measuring heart rate automatically

Many sports people prefer to use more convenient heart-rate monitors to measure heart beat. Basic models will simply measure heart rate, while more sophisticated models allow you to enter target heart-rate zones and view time spent under, in, and above the target zones after the session. Some computerized monitors allow you to download a training session for printing out. The basic set-up comprises a transmitter with an elasticated strap worn around the chest and a receiver resembling a watch worn around the wrist.

Determining your maximum heart rate

Maximum heart rate can be estimated from a simple calculation:

Maximum heart rate = 220 − age (years)

This calculation will give a *rough* idea of your maximum level. Everyone is different, however, so this approximation may not be terribly accurate. A more accurate and individual way is through a fitness test, perhaps at the gym, where you exercise to your own maximum level under the supervision of a qualified professional. You can also estimate this level in the self-assessment tests in Chapter 2 by taking your heart rate immediately at the end of the aerobic capacity test (12-minute run), the last 2 minutes of which you should run flat out. Read the chapter, do the questionnaires and take the precautions outlined at the beginning of the chapter first.

TRAINING LEVELS

Once you know your maximum heart rate (MHR) you will be able to calculate the percentages of this at which different sessions should be performed. Training can be broken down into 3 different levels:

1. Endurance pace   60-70% MHR
2. Steady pace   70-80% MHR
3. Threshold/intervals pace   80-90% MHR

Before you start any exercise programme, work out what your target heart rates will be for each of the 3 different kinds of training. You will end up with a range of heart rates for each level. To begin with you should aim for the lower end of this range.

Here is an example of a target heart rate calculation:

$$220 - age = MHR$$
or
$$220 - 25 \text{ (years)} = 195 \text{ bpm}$$

Calculate your own individual levels and insert them in the chart below.

Maximum heart rate = _____ beats per minute

Type of training	% MHR	Calculation	Range (bpm)
			Target Zone
Endurance	60-70	MHR × 0.6-0.7	_____ – _____
Steady	70-80	MHR × 0.7-0.8	_____ – _____
Threshold	80-90	MHR × 0.8-0.9	_____ – _____

Endurance-pace sessions

These are long, slow, distance training sessions conducted at a very comfortable pace at which you could carry on a conversation. They may seem as if you are not working hard enough but they are designed to increase the amount of blood and oxygen circulating (heart action) while placing minimum stress on the lungs. Don't be tempted to go faster in these sessions.

Steady-pace sessions

These will stress both the heart and lungs and involve working a little harder. This level is tougher and requires motivation to keep the pace going. You would get breathless if you tried to talk at this level.

Threshold- and intervals-pace sessions

These involve another step up, so that you are exercising at a pace at which lactic acid accumulates, giving you that tired and heavy legs/arms feeling. This type of session improves the efficiency of the lungs, which take in oxygen and transfer it to the blood, and also that of the muscles, which use fuel and oxygen. As the pace is difficult to maintain for extended periods, these sessions are broken down into intervals interspersed with recovery periods.

There is another intensity you can include or train at depending on your sport. This is your 'flat-out' or maximum pace that you can maintain for only short distances. There is no need to measure the heart rate during these bursts as you are required to put in your maximum effort. You must be in excellent condition before undertaking these, periodic, sessions.

So now you are equipped with your pace control. Don't worry if it all seems a bit laborious and time consuming as, after a while, you will get to know the feel of the different paces and zones and will not need to keep measuring.

Tips on heart rate

- As your fitness improves, your heart rate for each given level will decrease and you will find that you need to go faster to get up to the different HR levels. For example, on a very basic level, in week 1 you reach the lower end of your target zone with brisk walking but after a few weeks of training you will find that you need to jog to increase your heart rate sufficiently. This is because your efficiency has improved and more blood is being pumped per heart beat.

- Bear in mind that certain environmental factors will affect the heart rate response to exercise. In warm or humid conditions your heart rate may be higher than normal as the body has to work harder to get rid of the excess heat being generated by the muscles. If you are dehydrated you will also have an elevated heart rate, so remember to drink plenty before, during and after training.

CHAPTER 5

Resistance (Weight) Training

In our routine, non-active lives we generally possess enough muscular strength to complete tasks such as walking, running, lifting and so on. As we grow older, activities such as getting out of a chair can prove more difficult, which underlines the need for minimum strength levels for everyday functions.

Anyone doing a sport, whether socially, competitively or professionally, needs to be strong. And strength is improved through 'resistance training'. This means that the muscles are put under a load (resistance) which results in their becoming stronger, bigger or developing greater endurance. As we explained in Chapter 1, you can use your own body weight, elastic bands or other methods to apply resistance to the muscle(s). But the singular most effective method is weight training. Everybody, no matter what their sport, will benefit from weight training.

TYPES OF RESISTANCE (WEIGHT) TRAINING

Free weights (dumbbells and barbells)

Free weights are a cheap way of weight training – once you have bought them, you can use them for most muscle work. They also have the added advantage of enhancing the stability and strength of the joint as well as simply training the major muscles surrounding the joint. But correct lifting technique is vital when using free weights – you should really only consider their use at an intermediate to advanced level and make sure you get professional help and advice at a gym.

Remember that lifting heavy weights can cause injuries. So don't rely on your strength alone to stabilize your body when lifting free weights because if your technique is not perfect you could injure yourself. Gym machines avoid this risk of poor technique by 'fixing' the body in a stabilized position, enabling you to perform *only* the movement intended. For example, using a barbell to complete a standing biceps curl may encourage you to arch your back excessively, which can result in spinal problems if the weight is too heavy or if you become tired. A biceps curl machine or bench (preacher curl) won't let you lapse into poor technique.

Weight-training machines

There are basically two types of weight-training machine:

1. Variable-resistance equipment.
2. Accommodating-resistance equipment.

Variable-resistance equipment
Have you ever noticed how some exercises become easier at different points in the movement, as for instance in a free-weight biceps curl? This is due to the body's 'leverage' system which causes the tension in the muscles to change throughout a movement (one part being more difficult than another).

With variable-resistance equipment the *tension* in the muscle being used remains constant throughout the movement. It is called 'variable' because the machine changes the 'load' throughout to ensure that you feel a constant tension in your muscle. This results in a more even, and thus more effective, 'training effect'.

Variable-resistance equipment uses pulleys and cables to apply the resistance. Multi-station units (multi-gyms) are a good example of this type of equipment.

Accommodating-resistance equipment
A further development is accommodating-resistance equipment. You are unlikely to come across one of these machines as they are expensive and used generally in rehabilitation and medical settings. Where free weights and variable-resistance machines allow you to lift a weight at any speed you wish, accommodating resistance controls the *speed* of an exercise. Put simply, the faster you try to move, the more resistance the machine applies. These speeds can be set to achieve any training effect.

Static or isometric resistance

'Static' or 'isometric' resistance results in a build-up of tension in the muscle with no movement of the body. This is now a largely out-of-date method of training, though still used extensively in rehabilitation (and at one point by Charles Atlas!). Its disadvantage is that it improves strength only at the exact angle the limb is held. More importantly, it can significantly raise blood pressure above safe levels.

PRINCIPLES OF RESISTANCE TRAINING

So, in these types of weight training we see that there are four types of resistance:

1. Isometric or static resistance, where there is no movement.
2. Variable resistance, which produces a constant tension in the muscle.
3. Accommodating resistance, which also produces a constant tension in the muscle.
4. Constant resistance (free weights), where the tension in the muscle varies throughout the movement.

Now that you are all muscle-resistance experts, you can first plan your resistance training and then go on to look at some sample programmes and suggested exercises.

Any cursory glance at the growing number of fitness magazines will reveal thousands of different programmes and exercises for everything from healthy living to becoming Mr Universe. But the question is: 'What is right for me?' Don't worry. Now you know the theory of resistance training, you can understand anything you see or read on the subject. You can work out which type of resistance (1, 2, 3 or 4) will be occurring when you see an exercise. Now you need to know why certain programmes have specific effects.

Perfect Programming

If you want to be stronger, have better muscle endurance or become more powerful, what do you need to know and, more importantly, do?

1. A muscle will work harder and gain power only if it is 'overloaded' – that is, only if you push the muscle to do more than it can do currently will it improve. If you ask it to do something it is already

capable of, it will never improve. It must work until you can hardly work it any more. Scientists call this 'relative or complete temporary failure'. This temporary muscle failure is the only stimulus to ensure your muscle will improve.

2. If you wish to achieve the results shown below, try following the recommended number of sets and repetitions:

Desired result	Sets	Repetitions	Rest between exercise and set
pure strength	3-5	5-9	30 sec-1 min
strength and bulk	3-5	10-15	30 sec-1 min
mainly bulk	4-6	12-15	1-2 min
endurance	4-6	40-60+	30 sec-nil
power	2-4	3-5	4-5 min

3. *Specificity* is very important. There is little point in spending 80% of your training completing an exercise which is relevant to only 20% of your sport! This means that your exercises should mirror as closely as possible the types of movement you perform in your sport. Indeed, this is the biggest mistake made by sportsmen and women at every level.

> There is a classic story about a footballer who, because he didn't like sprinting, spent much of his training time in the pool and wondered why his sprinting was poor! Pool work would have been a reasonable off-season mode of training for stamina but was wholly inappropriate for developing leg speed in season.

4. If you don't use it, you lose it! All training, not just resistance training, is reversible. In season you will generally use your strength in training and playing and only 1 or 2 actual strength training sessions a week will be required.

Phases of play

Every resistance-training exercise has 2 distinct parts to the movement. Understanding these will help you get the best from every repetition. You'll also see how many other people never do!

45

Concentric and eccentric phases

Imagine lifting yourself out of a chair without using your arms. This action primarily uses the quadriceps (front thigh) and gluteal (backside) muscles. This lifting phase is called the *concentric* phase and uses contraction (shortening) of those muscles. Now, imagine lowering yourself back into the chair without using your arms. This also uses the quadriceps and gluteals but in a different way. This time the muscle is actually stretching (lengthening) from its shortest point in order to control your descent (although this may sound strange, it is what actually happens). This is called the *eccentric* phase of the movement. In resistance training, the eccentric phase is when you lower a weight. In any exercise the same muscle works both to lift (concentric) and lower (eccentric) the weight/resistance.

This is important to your training because you can get twice as much out of your training as those who don't realize how beneficial the eccentric phase is. It all comes down to speed.

Speed: slow down for strength

It's a common fault to overlook the speed of an exercise while placing the emphasis on how *much* you can lift. Remember that overload is needed to stimulate a muscle to grow. But it's not quite as simple as that. You achieve this overload by a combination of weight and speed. Because considerable resistance (weight = resistance) is required to produce 'overload', the concentric phase of an exercise will be slow, as no matter how hard you try, it's difficult to lift a very heavy weight quickly!

However, the eccentric phase (lowering) is generally given little thought and the resistance is often lowered at speed with little control. This is all well and good if you are using weights in circuit training or to improve muscle endurance (for, say, jogging) when you are looking to make the exercise as fast as possible, but with a good controlled movement.

But to get twice the benefit, slow down the eccentric phase of your movement to the same speed as the concentric. You may even slow it more than that. Eccentric phases may be 2 to 3 times longer and

In all exercises – apart from endurance training – try to achieve explosive movements in the concentric phase and slow movement in the eccentric phase, especially when power training with weights.

46

produce excellent gains, especially in stability strength around a joint. Such a slow lowering phase (superior eccentric strength) is especially effective as a precursor to explosive power training and is crucial to:

- developing jump height
- making an abrupt side-step
- developing the ability to stop on a dime!

Sports where this superior eccentric strength is invaluable are: javelin throwing, tennis/squash and most team sports.

MUSCLE-ENDURANCE TRAINING

Here, you are actually trying to move the weight as fast as possible yet with good control. Movements are more continuous and the speed of movement will be increased. You will be using lighter weights. This type of training is particularly useful for long-distance running.

PLANNING FOR PROGRESS

Don't forget to plan your training year (see Chapter 3). As in all training, in resistance training there are 3 divisions:

- recovery or rest period
- preparation period, consisting of 2 phases: (1) non-specific strength development, and (2) specific muscle development
- competitive period (not covered in this book).

Recovery period

During the recovery or rest period, activity is light and relatively infrequent. You will still be active, but let leisure and fun be your aim!

Preparation period

The preparation period is your most crucial and involves 2 distinct resistance-training phases. Lasting about 2 months this period coincides with the off-season and pre-season phases of the year and resistance training will usually span both of these phases. Divide your preparation-period resistance training into 2 distinct phases:

47

Phase 1: non-specific strength development

This is often called the 'gross' strength development phase.

Aim: To improve overall strength and, if required, put on muscle bulk.

What you do: A core set of exercises are used to develop your strength in the large, major muscles of the body. There are 7 key exercises. If you are not familiar with these, you should visit a gym and ask for tuition.

'Core' strengthening exercises		
Main body part affected	Entry level and endurance	Advanced level
chest/arms/shoulder	bench press machine	free-weight bench press
back/arms/shoulder	lateral pull down machine	seated rows
thighs/buttocks	leg press machine	dead lift or half squat
back of thigh	hamstring curl machine	hamstring curl machine
shoulders/neck	shoulder press machine	military press
overall		clean/clean and jerk
abdominals	various 'crunch' sit-ups	various 'crunch' sit-ups

Phase 2: specific muscle development

Now you will need to be far more specific in your resistance training. One phase will tend to merge into another and the new one will become increasingly dominant.

- If your sport demands that your muscles work at relatively low intensity for a long time, such as your legs in 10-km runs, you will move on to *muscle-endurance training*.
- On the other hand, if you are asked for explosive acceleration and hard physical contact, such as in rugby league or hockey, you would continue with *upper-body strength training* and use *power training* for your legs.

Some of the strongest sportsmen and women are not those who look the biggest but those who have diligently worked on their strength for 2, 3, 4, 5 or even 10 years. Be warned – if you don't use it, you'll lose it! If you stop training for 6 weeks or more, you will lose the strength you previously attained.

THE NUTS AND BOLTS OF CHANGE

If you have ever participated in resistance training, stopped for a few weeks and then resumed training, you will probably have noticed 3 things:

1. You will have been surprised at how quickly you made your initial gains.
2. You will have been appalled at how quickly your strength appeared to drop away.
3. Once you started training again, you will have surprised yourself by how quickly your old strength seemed to return.

There are 2 mechanisms at work here: crucial ones for you to get to grips with. When you use resistance training, both the muscle itself (structural components) and the nerves activating the muscles (neural components) are stimulated. Your initial improvement is due to neural factors: more muscle fibres (usually dormant) are being fired by the nervous system. At this point there is little structural change.

After 4-6 weeks the neural component is maximized and pure structural changes occur (the muscle tissue itself grows). Structural changes are long term, neural ones are relatively short. This explains why, when you stop training for a few weeks, there appears to be a disproportionate drop-off in strength. The improved 'structures' remain, just waiting to be activated again. This ensures that resistance-training gains made one year are not totally lost and can be built upon year on year.

FREQUENCY

So, how often should you use resistance training? Remember that any form of training is a stimulus towards growth, but it is the rest and recuperation time when growth actually occurs.

49

1. It takes a maximum of 36-48 hours for any muscle to recover from the overload you will apply to it in resistance training.
2. You must have a minimum of a day between training sessions.
3. You can train a muscle or muscle group only 3 times a week at most.

It is theoretically possible to train 4 times a week, on every other day: Monday, Wednesday, Friday, and then Sunday, Tuesday, Thursday, then Saturday, Monday, Wednesday, Friday, and so on. But this erratic schedule generally makes planning all other types of training such as aerobic, speed/acceleration and skill training very difficult and complex. Most athletes stick to a 2- to 3-session per week routine.

Entry level

You will make good gains in muscular development by following a twice-weekly routine for an initial 6-12 weeks. After this, resistance training 3 times a week will allow you to continue making gains. Three training sessions is the magic number for continual improvement. Additional sessions will provide little extra benefit, especially considering the extra time involved.

Advanced level

You require a strict 3 sessions per week to achieve on-going improvements. Once in your playing or competitive season, there is usually time for only 2 training sessions per week at best. This will be enough to maintain the work you have done and you will continue to see some improvement. The key, you will recall, is to ensure that your training intensity is high. In all but power training (see Chapter 7), keep your rest interval between each set short. A resistance-training session should take you no longer than 1-1¼ hours.

VARIETY

Without variation in your resistance-training programme, your body will quickly adapt to the demands of training and any improvement will be slow. The law of diminishing returns states that, as you train, gains and improvements will initially be high compared to the time committed. Over time, this rate of growth will diminish. This is true for all types of training. Vary the actual exercise, but keep a common theme such as power, strength or muscle endurance. Keep up 1 theme for 6-12 weeks. Although exercises may change (e.g. from bench press to dumbbell press for chest development), the basis of the training (low repetitions with long rest intervals between sets) must remain.

After the peak period of gains has been reached you should look to change radically the emphasis of your training. After 6 weeks of strength and bulk training, for example, try changing the type of training, e.g. from strength and bulk at 4-6 sets of 12-15 repetitions to muscle endurance training with 4-6 sets of 40 repetitions per set.

Periodically, have a 4- to 6-week break away from all resistance training. A good time to do this is at the beginning or mid-point in your competitive period. This allows your body some well-earned rest and recuperation, and often results in a sharp improvement in your game.

TYPES OF ROUTINE

There are essentially 2 types of resistance (weight)-training routine:

1. Those that follow scientific backing and work quickly and effectively.
2. Those that are a hybrid of the various scientific methods.

Providing you train hard enough for long enough, all resistance-training programmes will work. The key, of course, is to determine those that are the safest and most effective (see Chapter 3, which discusses the fundamentals upon which all programmes are based). Using that key, you will be able to determine the outcome and effectiveness of any programme.

The 3 basic types of training programme are:

1. Whole-body routines (opposing muscle groups).
2. Whole-body routines (pre-exhaustion).
3. Split routines.

Whole-body routines (opposing muscle groups)

These routines train all major muscle groups in the body in one training session.

Advantage: The most time-effective routines for athletes with several other components of fitness development also to consider. By progressively training the largest muscles, e.g. the thighs, and then the smaller muscles, e.g. the calves, you can ensure every major muscle is sufficiently stressed to elicit gains.

Working opposing muscle groups entails mixing your exercises so that no one area is worked repeatedly. For example, train legs first with a leg press or half squat and move on to a chest exercise such as the bench press. In this way, one muscle group has a small rest before it or the muscle group around it is stressed again. Use this approach if weight training is new to you. It still emphasizes the need to work to temporary muscle failure but in a manner which is less tiring (great for the psyche!). Use programme 1 below if you are just starting out. For someone returning to training after some time off or with a little experience, programme 2 is recommended.

Entry-level programme 1
Complete the exercises in order. What is your desired result? See the table on page 45 earlier in this chapter then do the sets and repetitions for that result.

Exercise	Body party affected
bench press	chest
half squat or leg press	legs/front
lateral pull down	back
hamstring curls	back of legs
seated rows	back
pec flys	chest
abdominal crunches	stomach

Entry-level programme 2

Exercise	Body part affected
half squat or leg press	front of legs
seated row	back
hamstring curl	back of legs
bench press	chest
tricep extensions	back of arms
shoulder press	back of arms/shoulders
lateral pull down	back
pec flys	chest
abdominal crunches	stomach

Advantage: time efficient. Try to complete your entire programme in 1-1¼ hours.

Since the initial gains made in muscular development are largely via the nervous system, with structural changes occurring some weeks later, the greater this neural input, the more stimulation there is to the muscle and, consequently, the greater your gains will be. In whole-body exercises, the entire nervous system is stimulated, particularly via the very large leg and buttock regions. This appears to heighten overall neural stimulation throughout the body, from which each exercise can benefit.

Whole-body routines (pre-exhaustion)

Unlike the opposing muscle-group routines, pre-exhaustion minimizes the muscles' rest and therefore produces greater overload in any one muscle or muscle group. To minimize this rest you work a muscle group first through an exercise that is 'compound', then through one that uses 'isolation'.

Compound exercises are those that, whilst targeting one large major muscle or muscle group, also allow you to utilize other muscles to assist in the movement. For example, the bench press aims at working your chest muscles (pectoralis major and minor), but considerable work is also achieved by the muscles in the back of the arms (triceps) and those of the front shoulder (anterior deltoid).

Isolation exercises aim to cut out, or at least reduce, those assisting muscle groups. An example is a pec fly (especially on a pec fly machine) which ensures that only your chest (pectoral) muscles are being worked.

Hence two consecutive exercises stress the same muscle group. A third exercise will often go on to work the assisting muscles from the first movement, i.e. in the case of the bench press, the back of the arms (triceps).

Remember, you are training for athletic development rather than to be a body builder. Unlike a body builder, who resistance trains for the sake of it and can spend many hours a day in the gym, you need to concentrate on several other aspects of your sport.

Here is an example of a pre-exhaustion advanced-level routine:

Exercise	Body part affected
bench press	chest, triceps, front shoulder
pec fly	chest
tricep extension	triceps
lateral pull down	back, biceps, back shoulder
seated row	back, biceps, back shoulder
reverse fly	back, some triceps
biceps curl	biceps
lateral raise	shoulders
half squat or leg press	buttocks, thighs
leg extensions	thighs
leg curl	hamstrings
abdominal crunches	stomach

For this routine, you need to be well organized. You need to move quickly between the exercises to maintain intensity throughout your training session. You should work to failure – i.e. push yourself to the point when you find it very difficult to complete another repetition or cannot complete another repetition.

You will notice that the abdominal exercises are always last. The abdominal muscle group is primarily responsible for stabilizing the trunk (movement sideways and forwards is a secondary role) and, as a consequence, is in constant use when you train in other exercises. If you exhaust this group too soon, you will find that the middle of your body is less stable and there is then an increased chance of injury as poor technique creeps into other exercises.

Split routines

As the name suggests, in these routines one group of muscles is trained one day and another on the next, and so on. These routines were first suggested by body builders who, spending large amounts of time in the gym, devised more elaborate routines.

As you know, to train muscles:

- overload should be applied and this overload should be progressive
- there should be sufficient rest to allow for growth
- there should be between 2 and 3 applications of the overload to the muscle per week.

Here is a typical training week if you are at a beginner's entry level or even a serious athlete in pre-season training:

Monday	resistance training
Tuesday	aerobic or speed training
Wednesday	resistance training
Thursday	aerobic or speed/acceleration training
Friday	resistance training
Saturday	rest day
Sunday	aerobic training

This example does not take into account team training, any pre-season competitions or warm-up games. Your training must, in many cases, be completed around your working day.

A typical split routine would look as follows:

Day 1	Chest Shoulders Triceps (abdominals)	usually 2-3 different exercises for one muscle group
Day 2	Back Legs Biceps (abdominals)	usually 2-3 different exercises for one muscle group

To meet the scientific requirements for improvement, you would need to train at least 4 days per week for 2 overload sessions per muscle group, and up to 6 times a week for 3 overload sessions per muscle group per week, using a split routine.

Clearly this leaves little time for any other training related to your activity. Indeed, other types of muscular training, such as strength training one day and acceleration training the next, can place maximum stress on the muscles and leave insufficient time for rest. Split routines, although in common use, are incompatible with a sports person's training as they require too much time in the gym. They are not suitable for full-time, professional athletes. In general, whole-body training routines are preferable and recommended.

CHAPTER 6

Flexibility Training

Flexibility is important in all sports because it will reduce the likeli-hood of injury, make specific movements smoother and allow you to get more power behind your shot! It is illustrated by the range of motions possible at a joint. There are 2 kinds of flexibility:

1. *Passive flexibility* is illustrated when a body part is relaxed then moved through its range of motion (or ROM) by another person.
2. *Dynamic flexibility* can be seen when the ROM at a joint is achieved through contractions of the muscles that control that joint.

Dynamic flexibility is the primary area of emphasis in sport. This ROM can be influenced by a number of either external or internal factors.

FACTORS INFLUENCING FLEXIBILITY

Temperature

Your ROM is usually lower in the morning than in the afternoon. This is not so much to do with the time of day but with the body's temper-ature (which is higher in the afternoons). Research has shown that

The greatest flexibility in both males and females is usually achieved in the early school years, up until around 12 years of age. Girls are generally more flexible than boys due to their bone struc-tures and this advantage appears to continue throughout life.

warming a body to 113°F increased dynamic flexibility by about 20% and cooling the body to 65°F decreased the ROM by 10-20%. Muscles and connective tissue (tissue that binds muscle and joint muscle to bone) become quite pliable when warm, resulting in this temporary increase in range of motion. Thus, warming a muscle (and accompanying stretching) reduces the chance of injury to muscle and connective tissue.

Specificity of stretching

As with most other training effects, such as those for improving strength and aerobic capacity, flexibility tends to be specific to a particular movement. This results in a joint having good ROMs in certain directions and below-average ranges in other directions, depending on the use of the body part and the stretches employed. This can often lead to muscular imbalances. For example, muscles used to generate a movement (say the quadriceps in runners) develop flexibility through stretches or movement patterns regularly used, while other muscles surrounding the joint become less flexible. Many stretches aim to correct the imbalance by concentrating on those muscles that are secondary to the activity (e.g. hip flexors and hamstrings in runners). This is not to say that the primary muscle moves do not also need to be stretched.

Body type and flexibility

Muscle mass (as often seen in body builders) is usually unrelated to flexibility. In fact, weight training can improve ROM when a full range of movement is used in an exercise. Only when the bulk is very great will it interfere with the range of motion at a joint. The amount of body fat, however, does correlate to ROM. This is especially so around the neck, trunk and hips. Individuals with an excess of body fat show decreases in ROM.

Inactivity and flexibility

Equally, and often when in combination with increases in body fat, inactivity will decrease flexibility. Having a limb in plaster demonstrates this perfectly. The inactivity or lack of adequate activity of a muscle surrounding a joint, or of the joint itself, is a significant contributor to poor flexibility.

Bone structure, connective tissue and muscle

These internal factors have the greatest influence on flexibility. The way bones come together at a joint greatly limits the range of motion at that joint. This is extremely variable: a joint such as the shoulder has few limitations, while at the elbow the bone directly prevents the joint from over-extending.

Connective tissue is tissue that binds muscle, organs and other structures in the body. This includes the tendons and ligaments in a joint, and the joint capsule (the ligamentous tissue enclosing a joint). These structures contribute around 45-50% of the range of motion at a joint. Muscle fascia (the covering-over muscle) contributes 35-40%, while 8% is contributed by the tendons and 2% by the skin tension. From this you will see that up to 50% of a joint's ROM is influenced by the boney structures of the joint.

Strictly speaking, flexibility is not limited by the muscle itself but by connective tissue such as fascia. However, this is still part of the muscle and could reasonably be termed 'muscle tightness' for practical purposes.

IMPROVING FLEXIBILITY

We can improve our flexibility by doing stretching exercises. When stretching, it is important to follow these key practices:

1. Ensure that you are warm before you begin stretching. This means you should complete some light aerobic activity such as jogging or cycling for 3-5 minutes. Only work at a very low level (about 40% effort).
2. Begin with easy movements and progress to those you find more challenging.

Justifying the benefits of flexibility training is, to many sports participants, more necessary than justifying running, rowing, other aerobic training or strength training. The benefits of these seem more readily apparent than flexibility training. However, sportsmen such as Linford Christie, Alan Shearer and Nick Faldo appreciate the value of good flexibility and how it has improved their speed, agility or swing.

---

3. Do not bounce in 'static stretching'. Hold the stretch in a position that gives you a stretch sensation but does not cause pain. It is important to push the muscle slightly. However, if you stretch too aggressively, the muscle will actually contract as a protective response. This, of course, means that you won't get an improvement in your flexibility. In fact, you'll achieve the opposite!
4. Hold your warm-up stretches for 10-20 seconds. These should be repeated 3-4 times for each stretch, or on each side of the body.
5. Your warm-down stretches are, as you now know, the most important in terms of developing flexibility. These stretches should be held for anywhere between 30 and 60 seconds each. Again, complete 3-4 on each side. For those of you with specific tightness – if, say, the left feels tighter than the right, or you feel tight in a specific area – place an emphasis on that area by completing 2-3 more repetitions of the stretch until you feel more balanced, or generally more supple.

Static stretching: core stretching programme

Static stretching is a safe and effective way to develop flexibility. It involves a muscle within its limits, albeit at the end of those limits. To perform these stretches, you should follow the key practices mentioned above. Below is the core stretching programme you should use for all activities: it will ensure that all the major muscles are ready for activity. In addition, there are sports-specific stretches mentioned within each sport. These should be completed over and above the core programme.

CORE STRETCHING PROGRAMME

Calf
Stand with both feet facing forward and one foot about 0.25-0.5 m in front of the other. The front leg should be bent and the back leg straight. Lean slightly forward so that the weight is on the front leg. Press the heel of the back leg towards the ground, ensuring that the toes point straight forward. Hold for 10-15 seconds and repeat on the other leg. Feel the stretch in the calf muscle.

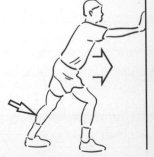

Achilles tendon

Stand with both feet facing forward and one foot about 0.25-0.5 m in front of the other. The front leg should be bent. Pull the back foot in slightly and bend the knee, shifting the weight to the back leg. Hold for 10-15 seconds and repeat on the other leg. Feel the stretch in the lower part of the calf and Achilles tendon.

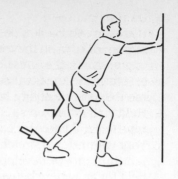

Hamstring

Stand with one foot raised on a bench, step or chair. Keep both legs soft at the knees and bend forward from the hips towards the raised foot. Look straight in front and keep the back straight. Hold and repeat with the other leg. Feel the stretch in the back of the thigh (hamstring).

Quadriceps

Stand with both legs together. Bend one leg up behind you and take hold of the ankle. Keep the knees together and hips facing forward, with the knee of the straight leg slightly bent. Hold and repeat with the other leg. Feel the stretch in the front of the thigh.

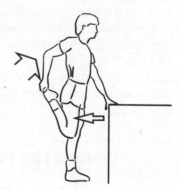

Front of hip

Step forward, bending your front leg and keeping your knee directly above the ankle. Stretch the other leg behind so that the leg is almost parallel to the floor. Rest your hands on the bent leg and keep the body straight. Press your hips forward and downward to stretch. Feel the stretch in the front of the hip of the back leg.

Lower back

Lie down on your back with your knees bent, feet flat on the floor and arms out to the sides at shoulder level. Rotate the knees to one side towards the floor, keeping the shoulder and upper body on the ground. Repeat with knees falling to the other side.

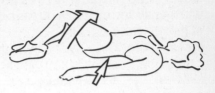

Chest and shoulder

Stand with the feet hip-width apart, facing a chair or bar. Lean forward, bending at the hips, to rest your hands on the chair. Relax the shoulders and drop your head between your arms. Feel the stretch across the arms, shoulders and back.

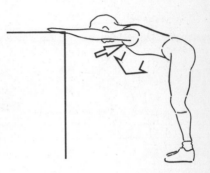

Dynamic stretching

Most sporting activities involve movement at speed, for example, a tennis swing of the arm or a kicking action of the leg in football. These actions require you to move a limb through its full ROM at speed. These dynamic movements stretch muscles and tendons aggressively and put them at some risk of injury if the movement goes beyond the limits of the joint range.

Dynamic stretching is appropriate particularly to sports that involve these fast, dynamic ballistic movements. In the warm-up, and after good static stretching, some dynamic movements may be of benefit to the advanced athlete. The movements always stay within the ROM of a joint – they just move through this range at speed, taking the form, for example, of high leg kicks or dynamic arm and trunk swinging. Dynamic stretching does not improve flexibility to any greater degree than static stretching. It may help in preparing the muscles and nervous system for what you are about to ask them to do in 'real' play, but it is important to note that dynamic stretching carries an element of risk, is useful only when warm, and should only be used by the advanced athlete.

Below are some of the more common dynamic stretching movements. Once you are well stretched from static stretching, begin these with gently flowing movements before increasing the force and speed of movement.

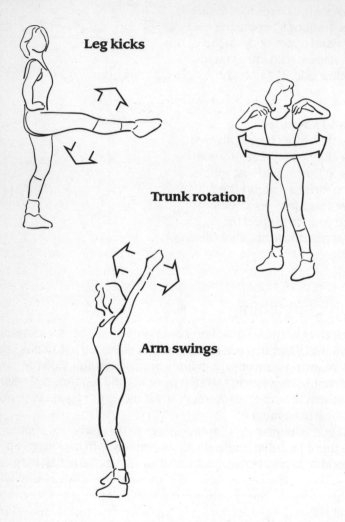

Leg kicks

Trunk rotation

Arm swings

CHAPTER 7

Plyometrics
(Developing Power, Acceleration and Jump Height)

In your sport, the ability to accelerate off the mark, jump to gain height or distance and move with power is very important. Plyometrics are effective in developing these abilities.

When a load is applied to a muscle, the muscle is stretched. In response to this rapid stretch the muscle immediately contracts (shortens) as a reflex action is initiated by the primary sensory receptor in the muscle – the muscle spindle. The muscle spindle detects both the magnitude and rate of charge (speed) in the length of muscle fibres. Applying a rapid stretch (through bouncing, jumping, etc.) to a muscle causes it to contract with greater force than normal. This contraction of the muscle generates considerable power, ideal for improving acceleration and jumping ability so vital to most sporting activities.

The word 'plyometric' comes from the Greek word *pleythyein*, meaning 'to increase', or from the Greek roots *plio* and *metric*, meaning 'more' and 'measure'. Plyometric movement is based on the reflex contraction of muscle fibres as a result of rapid loading and stretching of those fibres. Expressed another way, plyometrics can be thought of as *stretch-shortening cycles* of a particular muscle or muscle fibres.

> Considerable stress is involved in practising any form of bouncing, jumping or hopping. Consequently, you must ensure you are completely free from injury before using plyometric exercises. It is very important that you begin with a low number of exercises and repetitions.

TECHNIQUE GUIDELINES

For plyometric movement to be effective and safe you must:

- Always warm up and cool down thoroughly. Because the exercises are so explosive, it is vital that you are fully stretched and warm.
- Ensure that you have the motor skill necessary to perform the exercises you use. That is, you should be able to bound, hop and jump easily.
- Remember to perform at your maximum level of intensity to gain from plyometrics.
- Make your movements explosive.
- Ensure that you generate the maximum force you can in each movement.
- Minimize the contact time on the ground, i.e. your foot should spend as little time in contact with the ground as possible.

The overload you apply must be gradual yet progressive. As in resistance training, too great a load is detrimental unless your form remains perfect. Increase the number of repetitions slowly, emphasizing the speed of movement.

Rest is vital. The exercises are exceptionally demanding and it is important to rest for at least 48-72 hours between training sessions. One training session per week is adequate when you begin, and never do more than 2-3 sessions per week.

Other technique guidelines

1. Foot (feet) placement is very important when performing the drills. Whenever possible, stay on the ball of your foot. This can be very difficult. Although a flat-foot landing is acceptable, it is better to land on the ball of the foot. In either case, the ankle/foot should be locked in position so that no rolling occurs.

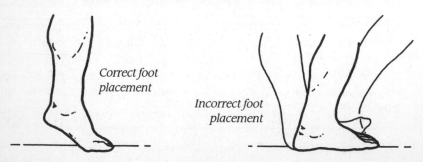

Correct foot placement

Incorrect foot placement

When performing plyometrics, use only body weight as there is nothing more to be gained and a very significant increase in risk of injury if you use additional weight such as weighted vests, dumbbells, bars, and so on.

2. It is important to maintain a 'knees-up', 'thumbs-up' position in all jumps, bounds, hops, etc. This keeps your body balanced and helps to ensure your foot lands in a straight line rather than splayed out. Additional power is also generated in this position as the tendency to drop the shoulders forward is decreased.

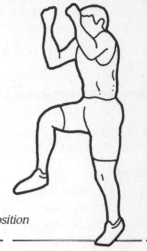

A knees-up, thumbs-up position

3. Remember that the whole basis of plyometrics is the speed of movement. The transitions between the 'yielding' phase and the 'overcoming' phase (in jumping, the 'landing' and 'rebounding' phases) should be as fast as possible. To ensure this, make your landings as undamped as possible. Damped landings reduce the release time and thus the effectiveness of the exercise. Use a firm surface with some give, but not an excessive amount. Sprung wooden floors, grass and good running tracks are ideal. Your footwear must be supportive and in good repair.

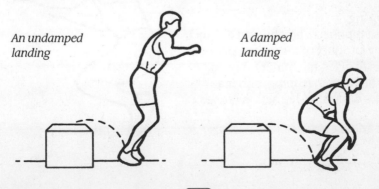

An undamped landing

A damped landing

ENTRY-LEVEL EXERCISES

While there is a range of upper-body plyometric exercises involving swings, throws and twists, they are limited in their application. This section will concentrate on lower-limb plyometrics which will increase leg power, and off-the-mark acceleration (speed) and jump-height ability. The exercises are made up of a series of leaps, hops, jumps and ricochets.

Leaping
Leaping is a one-off effort where maximum height and distance are attempted. Leaps can be executed with both legs or on a single leg.

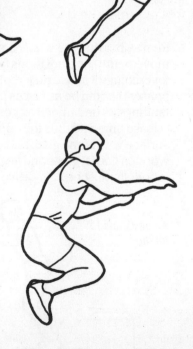

Skipping
Skips are performed as a series of hops, alternating the legs and taking a skip or step between each hop. Again, the emphasis should be on distance covered and height achieved.

Hopping
Hops emphasize height, and distance is a by-product of these movements. The rate of leg movement is usually very high. As in leaping, either a single- or double-leg action is used.

Jumping

Jump exercises aim to achieve maximum height. Ground contact time is longer as the knees bend further but the movement should still be executed as fast as possible. Distance is not of concern. Use either one or both legs.

Ricochets

Ricochets are a series of very rapid foot movements. Stay on the toes (ball of the foot) and emphasize the speed of movement. Minimize the height and distance covered.

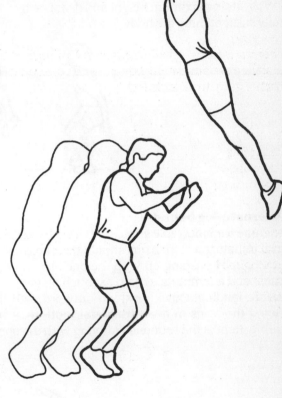

ADVANCED-LEVEL EXERCISES

In conjunction with fundamental skips, hops, jumps and ricochets there is a series of more advanced exercises which increase the load on the muscle. Recent research suggests that speed of movement is more important than the magnitude of the load in increasing acceleration and jumping ability. Whatever exercise you are performing, speed is essential. The following exercises are recommended for developing leg power.

Double-leg bound

Begin the exercise from a half-squat stance. Arms should be down at the sides, with shoulders forward and out over the knees. Keep the back straight and hold the head up. Jump outward and upward, using the extension of the hips and forward thrusting movement of the arms. Try to attain maximum height and distance by fully straightening the body.

Alternate-leg bound

Assume a comfortable stance with one foot slightly ahead of the other as if initiating a step. Arms should be relaxed at the sides.

Begin by pushing off with the back leg, driving the knee up to the chest and attempting to gain as much height and distance as possible before landing. Quickly extend outward with the driving leg. Either swing the arms in a contralateral motion or execute a double-arm swing. Repeat the sequence (driving with the opposite leg) on landing.

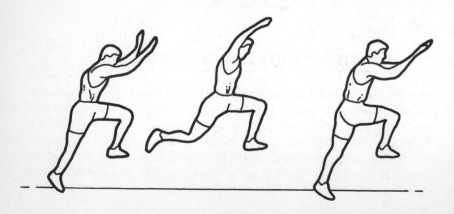

Incline bound

This is performed as for the double-leg bound but at the bottom of a hill of no greater than 20 degrees incline. Explode upwards from step to step, gradually increasing the number of steps or distance. Use the arms in an upward thrusting motion to help achieve the upward lifting action.

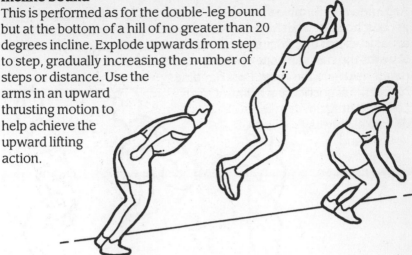

Double-leg speed hop

Assume a relaxed stance with a straight back, head up and shoulders slightly forward. Keep arms at sides and bend at 90 degrees with the thumbs up. Begin by jumping upward as high as possible, flexing the legs completely so as to bring the feet under the buttocks. Emphasize maximum lift by bringing the knees high and forward with each repetition. On each landing, jump quickly upwards again with the same cycling action of the legs, using the arms to achieve maximum lift. The action sequence should be executed as rapidly as possible. Work at gaining height and distance, but not at the expense of repetition rate.

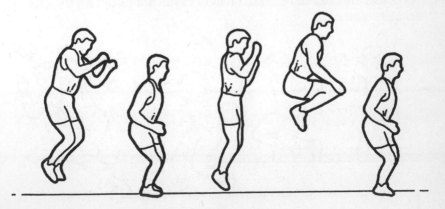

Knee-tuck jump

Assume a comfortable upright stance, placing the hands palms down at chest height. Begin by rapidly dipping down to about the quarter-squat level and immediately explode upward. Drive the knees high towards the chest and attempt to contact the knees to the palms of the hands held near the chest. Upon landing, repeat the sequence, each time concentrating on driving the knees upward and tucking the feet under the body.

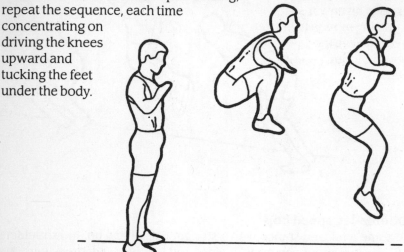

Side-jump sprint

Place cones 14-19 m in front of the starting point to act as a finish line. Stand on one side of a bench, facing the start line, with feet together. Begin by jumping sideways back and forth over the bench for 2 repetitions. On landing on the last jump, explode forward into a sprint to the finish line. Anticipate the landing and be ready to sprint forward. Emphasis should not be on the height of the jumps but on the rate of acceleration.

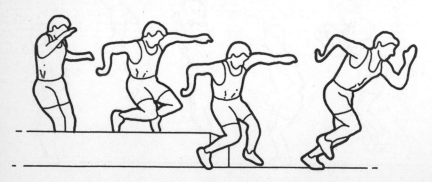

Double-leg box bound

With boxes spaced evenly 1-2 m apart, stand approximately 2-3 steps in front of the first box. Feet should be slightly more than shoulder-width apart. The body is held in a semi-squat stance with the back straight, head up and arms at sides. Begin by exploding upward on to the first box. As soon as you land on the box, explode upward again as high and as far out as possible, landing on the ground. Repeat the sequence until completed.

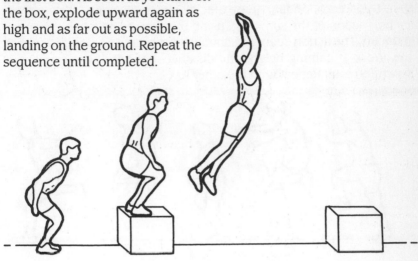

Alternate-leg box bound

Assume the same stance as in the alternate-leg bound exercise described above, 2-3 steps in front of a series of boxes spaced approximately 1-2 m apart. The action sequence is as for the alternate-leg bound (see page 68) except that every step is made from a box.

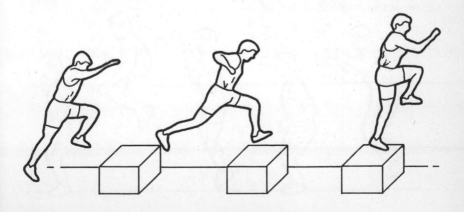

Single-leg speed hop

Assume a relaxed stance with a straight back, head up and shoulders slightly forward. Keep arms at sides and bend at 90 degrees with the thumbs up. Begin by jumping upward as high as possible, flexing one leg completely so as to bring the foot under the buttocks. Emphasize maximum lift by bringing the knee high and forward with each repetition. Upon each landing, jump quickly upwards again with the same cycling action of the same leg, using the arms to help achieve maximum lift. The action sequence should be executed as rapidly as possible. Work at gaining height and distance, but not at the expense of repetition rate. Repeat with the other leg.

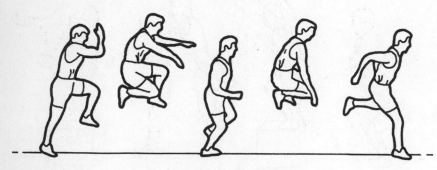

Incremental vertical jump

Suspend a rope in a taut line between 2 points, about 0.3-1 m above the ground (depending on your height), with one end nearer the ground than the other. Assume a relaxed position immediately to the side of the lowest end of the rope with feet together. Jumping back and forth over the rope, try to advance up the rope as high as possible. Bring the knees forward and upward towards the chest whilst tucking the feet underneath the buttocks. Continue up the rope as far as possible, thus completing the set.

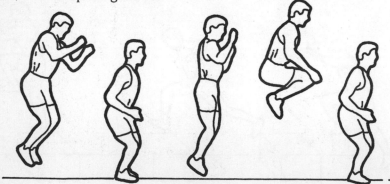

Skipping

Assume a relaxed standing position with one leg slightly in front of the other. Driving off with the back leg, initiate a short skipping step. Then thrust the opposite leg to chest level and repeat the action with the opposite leg on landing. A pattern of right-right-step-left-left-step-right-right is executed. Obtain as much height and explosive power as possible on each skip. Drive the knee and arms as high as possible, concentrating on 'hang-time' (time spent in the air between jumps). Minimize the time spent on the ground.

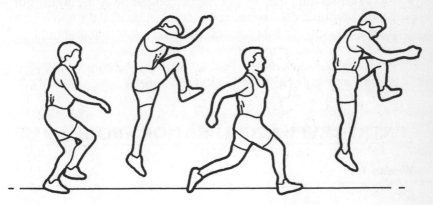

Two-box bound

Place two 45-cm boxes approximately ½ m apart. Stand on the first box in a comfortable stance with feet shoulder-width apart. Jump off box 1 and recoil off the floor on to box 2. Turn around and repeat the exercise back the other way.

There and back is one repetition.

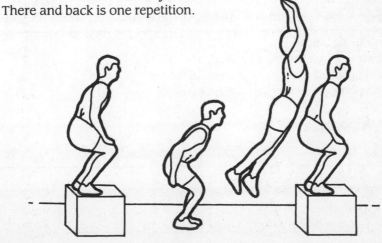

Points to note for advanced exercises

- Boxes should be of a sturdy design and capable of supporting not only the resting body weight but body weight landing on top of them. They should be no more than 45 cm in height. This has been shown to be ideal for retaining maximum contact time while supplying sufficient magnitude.
- Hopping, skipping, bounding and ricochet distances should be no more than 15 m.
- It is vital to ensure that, in any one training session, the number of ground contacts does not exceed 250. That is, of all the hops, jumps, bounds, etc. that you complete, your foot or feet should touch the ground no more than 250 times. Although the programmes below ensure this, the total ground contact will vary slightly as people have varying jump distances.

ENTRY-LEVEL ACCELERATION PROGRAMME

Weeks 1-2

Exercise	Distance/repetitions	Sets
double-leg bound	over 10 m × 6	2
ricochets	over 10 m × 6	2
single-leg speed hop	over 10 m × 6	1

Weeks 3-4

Exercise	Distance/repetitions	Sets
alternate-leg bound	over 10 m × 8	2
alternate-leg box bound	8 reps	2
single-leg speed hop	over 15 m × 8	2
two-box bound	8 reps	2

Week 5 onwards

Exercise	Distance/repetitions	Sets
two-box bound	10 reps	3
ricochets	over 15 m × 8	2
incline bound	over 10 m × 8 (low angles only)	2
single-leg speed hop	over 15 m × 10	2

ADVANCED-LEVEL ACCELERATION PROGRAMME

Weeks 1-2

Exercise	Distance/repetitions	Sets
ricochets	over 15 m × 8	2
alternate-leg bound	over 15 m × 8	2
double-leg speed hop	over 15 m × 8	2

Weeks 3-4

Exercise	Distance/repetitions	Sets
two-box bound	10 reps	2
alternate-leg box bound	10 reps	3
single-leg speed hop	over 15 m × 10	2
side-jump sprint	10 reps	2

Week 5 onwards

Exercise	Distance/repetitions	Sets
ricochets	over 10 m × 6	1
alternate-leg bound	over 10 m × 6	1
two-box bound	10 reps	2
side-jump sprint	10 reps	2
single-leg speed hop	over 10 m × 8	2
skipping	over 10 m × 8	2

Pre-pubescent athletes and adolescents can gain valuable physical attributes, such as co-ordination and muscular development, from the overloads provided by plyometrics. However, it is vital that all participants have the base strength to cope with the exercise loads. Clearly, these types of movement are natural activities which children and adolescents perform every day. But emphasis must be on technique of the highest standard. Training intensities must be low with plenty of rest between sets. All sets and repetitions should be halved for young athletes, who should begin at one-third of the recommended amount.

ENTRY-LEVEL JUMP PROGRAMME

Weeks 1-2

Exercise	Distance/repetitions	Sets
knee-tuck jump	10 reps	4
skipping	over 10 m × 6	2
incremental vertical jump	over 10 m × 6	2

Weeks 3-4

Exercise	Distance/repetitions	Sets
double-leg bound	over 10 m × 8 (emphasize height)	3
double-leg box bound	10 reps	3
alternate-leg box bound	10 reps	3

Week 5 onwards

Exercise	Distance/repetitions	Sets
incline bound	over 10 m × 6	1
incremental vertical jump	over 10 m × 6	2
knee-tuck jump	10 reps	3
alternate-leg bound	10 reps	3

ADVANCED-LEVEL JUMP PROGRAMME

Weeks 1-2

Exercise	Distance/repetitions	Sets
double-leg bound	10 reps	2
incline bound	over 15 m × 8	2
double-leg box bound	10 reps	3
knee-tuck jump	10 reps	3

Weeks 3-4

Exercise	Distance/repetitions	Sets
incline bound	over 15 m × 10	3
double-leg bound	10 reps	3
incremental vertical jump	over 15 m × 10	3
alternate-leg bound	10 reps	3

Week 5 onwards

Exercise	Distance/repetitions	Sets
knee-tuck jump	10 reps	3
incremental vertical jump	over 10 m × 8	2
alternate-leg box bound	10 reps	3
double-leg bound	10 reps	3
incline bound	over 10 m × 10	2
double-leg speed hop	over 10 m × 10	2

SAFETY PRECAUTIONS

Plyometrics can make a considerable difference to your speed, acceleration and jump height. But there are risks. This sort of training is very advanced and demands good strength, flexibility and aerobic levels before undertaking. Make sure you rest for 4-5 minutes between each set of an exercise and that, during this time, you stretch gently. If at any time you feel any degree of pain or uncommon discomfort, stop immediately and discontinue that session. Such are the loads (magnitudes and speeds) that you cannot train on even the slightest injury, or continue to train if you slightly 'tweak' a muscle. Having said all of this, plyometrics are an effective way of making some quite staggering gains. Just remember to approach these exercises with care.

CHAPTER 8

Team Sports

FOOTBALL

Football is a multiple-sprint sport involving short bursts of high-speed activity interspersed with periods of lower-intensity walking or jogging.

What determines good play in football?

- speed
- acceleration
- endurance to recover from high-speed bursts and to last the whole game (90 minutes, excluding extra time).

Periods of rest and recovery are unpredictable and variable, dictated by the pattern of play and how spontaneous you are. The speed and demands of the game will largely depend on the level of competition that you play at. The skills involved include:

- the ability to work with a team
- running, kicking, shooting, passing and controlling the ball at speed
- tackling
- the capacity to rapidly change direction.

Football players are prone to poorer hamstring flexibility than non-players or even non-exercisers. This could reflect a lack of attention to flexibility in training (is this you?).

Indoor football

Typically a 5-a-side game, indoor football is more intense, slightly faster, and does not last as long as 'outdoor' football. The differences in physical demands between the various positions are minor except for those between the goalkeeper and the rest of the team. Winning teams can blend all the individual characteristics into a coherent playing machine.

HOW STRENUOUS IS FOOTBALL?

During a game, a player may cover up to 10 km through a combination of walking, jogging, running and sprinting, with an average speed of 7 km per hour. The pattern of play in league games has been studied and shown to consist of almost 1000 bouts of action incorporating rapid and frequent changes in speed and direction. The average burst lasts about 6 seconds and covers about 15 m, but there is a huge difference from one extreme to the other. The higher the level of competition, the shorter and fewer the rest periods – you have to run faster and have less time to recover.

Heart rates

Players exercise at about 80% of their maximum heart rate. So, the better your aerobic capacity, the higher the intensity you will be able to maintain during a game. Although the game is varied in pace and intermittent in nature, your heart rate does stay at a fairly high level throughout.

Energy

If you play a 90-minute game at a moderate pace you would burn up about 588 kilocalories, or about 1.2 kilocalories per minute. The exact amount of calories varies according to your individual body weight. See the table in Appendix 2 to determine the energy use based on your body weight. The energy demands of football increase according to the amount of time you spend on the ball, so it's important in training that you spend a fair amount of your time running with the ball at set speeds, as well as in straightforward running.

At international level, energy demands can be as high as 13 kilocalories a minute with a total expenditure for the game reaching almost 1200 kilocalories.

PLAYER PROFILE: ENTRY LEVEL

People of all ages play recreational football, but the average age is 25-35 years. You can, of course, continue playing for many years beyond this – the pace of the game and the amount of contact and tackling will suit your abilities if you play with others of a similar fitness level. Note that veterans' football has its own league! The player profile and level of fitness differ vastly depending on whether you play football once or twice a month and do little or no other exercise, or whether you play every week with other activities thrown in to increase your fitness for football.

Your size and shape

Footballers come in all heights and weights. But as it is a weight-bearing sport you should keep body fat and weight down to relieve stress on your joints, particularly the knees. Extra fat is also 'dead' weight and will slow you down. Strength in the quadriceps and hamstrings (the front and back of the thigh) is above average in footballers.

Aerobic capacity and heart rate

Aerobic capacities of footballers, as measured by VO_2 max, are in the range of 45-55 ml/kg/min in recreational players and are fairly easy to achieve through regular aerobic training. Resting heart rate tends to be around 60 bpm as a good recovery rate is important between fast bursts.

PLAYER PROFILE: ADVANCED LEVEL

Professional footballers tend to have a playing career of about 10 years, playing at their peak level for about 5 years. The average age is about 25 years with some players continuing into their 30s (some goalkeepers play professionally up to 40 years of age).

Your size and shape

The heights and weights of advanced-level football players vary enormously. Physical shape tends to go hand-in-hand with choice of playing position. For the goalkeeper, height tends to be an advantage for obvious reasons. Leg strength is highly important for effective turning, kicking and changing pace, while upper-body strength is useful for throw-ins and heading (a strong neck).

PLAYER PROFILE: ALL PLAYERS

Problem areas

Two common physical problem areas often found in football players can make them prone to certain types of injury and need to be taken into account:

- an imbalance between the quadriceps at the front of the thigh and the hamstrings at the back
- a strength imbalance between the right and left leg.

Aerobic capacity and heart rate

A well-developed, high anaerobic capacity is absolutely essential to play a good, pacey game and to repeat fast bursts of running. The average maximum aerobic capacity (VO_2 max) for international and top league players ranges between 55-70 ml/kg/min. Note that aerobic capacity varies depending on the stage in the training or competitive season. Goalkeepers tend to have lower levels and active midfield players the highest. The resting heart rate of most advanced players tends to be around 52-62 bpm and between 48-52 bpm in top league and international players.

To summarize, these are some of the specific fitness levels important in football:

- good muscle development and strength geared towards fast movements
- low level of body fat
- excellent aerobic and anaerobic capacity for acceleration, speed and a good recovery rate
- low resting heart rate.

TRAINING PHASES

Football demands both physical and technical skills, and these need to be incorporated into the training plan. The training year for anyone playing regular club, amateur or professional football can be broken up into different phases.

1. *Off-season*. The off-season phase is the period between the end of the previous season (last game) and the first game of the new season. In the first month you should aim to maintain fitness through other sports or activities.

2. *Pre-season*. The pre-season phase marks the return to regular and targeted training. At first, the focus is usually on improving basic fitness, stamina and strength; later the emphasis is on match-specific fitness, incorporating some technical and skill work through drills and match-type situations.

3. *During the season*. Once the season starts you need to maintain your aerobic fitness through running and interval training but time can be limited if you are playing regular games. There is a trade-off between skill and fitness training, but doing interval work with the ball and against opposition can incorporate both aspects.

ENTRY-LEVEL TRAINING

Trying to develop fitness 'as you go' can lead to injury or excessive stiffness. It is important you achieve a basic degree of fitness before you play. What physical attributes do you need, as a recreational or occasional player? A 'good engine' is essential. In other words, a reasonable degree of aerobic stamina (the ability to 'run all day'). Aerobic fitness is fundamental to all players, and even goalkeepers will benefit from aerobic stamina to aid concentration over long periods of inactivity. Running is the best kind of aerobic training, but cycling can be used as an alternative and 25% of the effect can be achieved through other aerobic activities such as swimming, or using rowing or step machines.

Advantages of aerobic training

- Increases your capacity to perform at a higher intensity (pace) for a longer time, and thus your ability to move to the ball more frequently, make runs more easily and undertake faster transitions from offence to defence.
- Minimizes the number and severity of potential injuries and helps you to become more resistant to fatigue which can cause loss of concentration and co-ordination.
- Increases your ability to recover from high-intensity practice sessions and from games.

Developing aerobic capacity

Duration

To see any improvement from training you need to work for a certain period of time. Duration can be expressed either in time or distance, but both are linked. For example, if during your initial training you can run 5 km in 20 minutes you will want to improve on this time as your fitness improves. Always link distance to time to gauge improvements.

For running, follow the chart below for safe progress in the early stages of your aerobic training.

Week	Duration (min)	Terrain
1-2	15-20	flat, soft surface, grass, etc.
3-4	20-30	flat or undulating mixed surfaces
5-6	30-40	moderate incline hills, mixed surfaces

Frequency

One run a month is not going to do you much good. But 10 runs a week will be just as bad! Ideally, run 3 times a week. If you are starting from a very low level of fitness begin with 2 runs a week. If you are already in training you should try to run a maximum of 4 times a week.

Intensity

Once you have determined the frequency and duration of each run, you must determine the 'intensity' (how hard) your runs should be. It is important to work to a pre-determined intensity for several reasons. Working at the same intensity on every run will limit the benefits you can achieve. But if you work within a specific range of intensity you will gain good aerobic stamina. A range of between 60-75% of your maximum heart rate (MHR), discussed in detail in Chapter 4, will allow you to determine your exact training intensity.

For the example given in the table above we recommend you follow 3 training intensities:

Duration (min)	Intensity (% of MHR)	
15-20	week 1: 60	week 2: 65-70
20-30	week 3: 70	week 4: 75
30-40	week 5: 60-70	week 6: 70-75

Maintaining the correct training intensity ensures that the appropriate training effect is achieved. Many athletes, even at world-class level, mistakenly believe 'more is better'. Training above 75% MHR will have a different effect on your heart, lungs and muscles than the one we are looking to achieve here. You will need to train at a higher intensity (speed) in the pre-season part of your training, but not at the moment.

Strength training

Superior leg strength enhances your power, speed and acceleration. Good upper-body strength ensures that you can better hold an opponent off the ball and compete in contact situations. Chapter 5 shows you how to gain maximum benefits from resistance (strength) training. At an entry level, it is best to train at a low intensity until you are technically proficient and your muscles and joints are accustomed to the loads.

Here is a strength-training programme for entry level.

Exercise	Sets	Repetitions	Rest between sets	Load
half squat or leg press	3-5	5-9	30 sec-1 min	80-85% of your maximum ability
leg curl	3-5	5-9	30 sec-1 min	80-85% of your maximum ability
bench press	3-5	5-9	30 sec-1 min	80-85% of your maximum ability
lateral pull down	3-5	5-9	30 sec-1 min	80-85% of your maximum ability
shoulder press	3-5	5-9	30 sec-1 min	80-85% of your maximum ability
abdominal crunches	3-5	20-40	30 sec-1 min	body weight

Complete the exercises in order and remember to give the muscles time to recover and grow. Training is merely the stimulus for improvements which take place during rest. For optimum results, complete the above routine every other day.

Developing speed and acceleration

Sprinting from a standing/walking start or running at top pace for a period of time (such as a long-ball run) requires you to use the anaerobic system (see Chapter 1). This type of training is very demanding so you must first build a good level of strength, flexibility and aerobic endurance. Once you have completed 6 weeks of aerobic training, and have improved your strength and flexibility, you will be ready to develop specific football fitness.

By watching games at your level you will be able to judge how far and what 'shape' your sprinting takes. A right back, for example, will complete many runs to the right, an equal number of lateral moves to the left when defending and maybe up to 10-20 diagonal runs in a number of directions. Your sprint drills should mirror these patterns of running. In this example, the player sprints from cone to cone in a number of different directions and with a variety of sprinting styles.

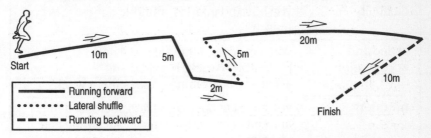

An example of a sprint drill, showing the runner running in different directions and in different styles

To get the best gains follow the programme below, ensuring you change the drill pattern (direction) after each set. Make the patterns as realistic as you can, based on the level you play at:

Repetitions per set	Number of sets	Rest between sets (min)
3	2-3	5
6	3	4
8-10	2-3	1-2

Remember that you should give each set and repetition your maximum effort. Walk back to the start as your rest between each repetition and stretch between each set.

TRANSITION GOALS

To successfully complete your fitness training and to ensure that you are physically ready to move on to the advanced training, it is important that you can first reach some minimum safety and fitness levels. Below are the transition goals you should be able to complete before attempting the advanced-level training section for football.

Component	Goal
aerobic capacity	you have completed 80% of the first 6 weeks' training
strength	you have completed all of the first 6 weeks' training (i.e. trained every other day excluding Saturdays and Sundays) for 6 weeks
flexibility	you have no injuries or undue tightness in any muscle
speed and acceleration	you have completed at least 4 and preferably 6 weeks of speed and acceleration training – 2 sessions a week
nutrition	you have cut back on all fats, increased the amount of carbohydrate you are eating (see Chapter 11) and are drinking at least 4-8 glasses of water a day

ADVANCED-LEVEL TRAINING

Having reached your transition goals for each of the areas defined above, you are now ready to undertake more demanding training.

The weekly schedule

At this level you will benefit from sticking to a more structured programme, one that will allow training twice a day. This will be easier if you are a semi-professional/professional player, but as an amateur you may be surprised how some good organization on your part can make it possible to fit a twice-daily routine around your work commitments.

Those of you lucky enough to be able to train twice a day should follow these recommended guidelines:

	Session 1	Session 2
Mon	strength	long aerobic run
Tues	rest	speed & acceleration
Wed	strength	long aerobic run/cycle, etc. or circuit
Thurs	speed & acceleration	rest
Fri	strength or rest	light aerobic session or rest
Sat	rest	rest or game
Sun	rest	light swim, jog, cycle & stretch

Those able to train only once a day should follow these guidelines:

Mon	strength
Tues	speed & acceleration
Wed	strength
Thurs	long aerobic run or circuit
Fri	strength or rest
Sat	rest or game
Sun	light aerobic session & stretch

There will be individual differences in the training you can complete depending on the number of games you play each week, time spent travelling to games and team training sessions that must be completed around your personal-fitness development work. Three rules should be followed when you devise your specific training week:

1. Always rest the day before and morning of a game (a very light team run-out is OK).
2. Never train the same component (speed, strength, etc.) twice in a row. Take 24 hours' rest between identical types of training. This doesn't mean you can't train in other areas, particularly stretching.

3. Never train on an injury. However, you should not stop training when injured, but train around the injury by swimming, cycling, or doing upper-body strength training.

Aerobic training

Wherever possible, try to train at least once a week by running. As fitness improves, you will find it increasingly difficult to reach the correct training heart rate through other activities such as swimming or biking. Running is also very specific to the game, so it is ideal for your aerobic fitness. Follow the guidelines below:

Week	Duration (min)	Terrain	Intensity (% of MHR)
1-3	20-30	mixed soft	80%
4-6	40-50	surfaces but	80%
7-12	30-50	with hills	75-85%

Circuit training (see diagram opposite)

To complement your aerobic training (not to replace it!) circuit training is a very productive workout. Work to the same training guidelines as for aerobic training above. For each exercise and the number of exercises in the circuit vary the number of times you complete the circuit, the number of repetitions or the time you exercise at each station. This keeps the variety up and ensures you train to the right duration.

When using circuits it is important that you vary the running distances and directions in each training session. This encourages ongoing improvements and challenges your ability to design training routines to match your game! After you have become familiar with a circuit, it is worthwhile training with a ball on some of the laps. This allows for a skill component to be introduced which enhances your ability to run, turn and move with the ball.

Strength (resistance) training

Resistance training will bring enormous benefits to your game. As you become stronger you do not necessarily have to become more muscular. Increased muscle bulk (known as muscle hypertrophy) is possible but is not always required. Improving pure tensile strength,

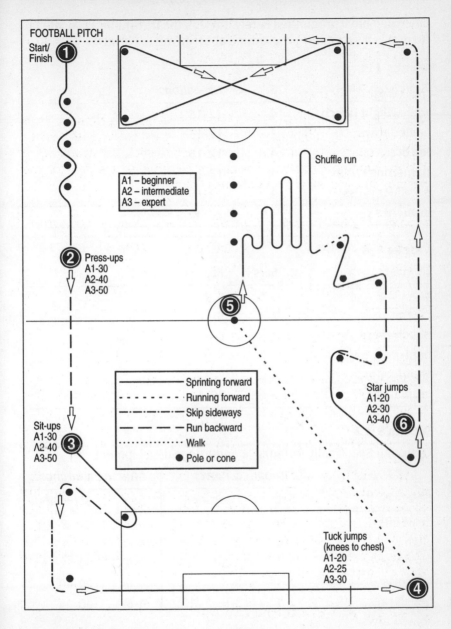

FOOTBALL PITCH

Start/
Finish ①

② Press-ups
A1-30
A2-40
A3-50

A1 – beginner
A2 – intermediate
A3 – expert

Shuffle run

⑤

Sit-ups
A1-30
A2 40
A3-50 ③

——————— Sprinting forward
· · · · · · · · · Running forward
·—·—·—·— Skip sideways
— — — — Run backward
· · · · · · · · · Walk
● Pole or cone

Star jumps
A1-20
A2-30
A3-40 ⑥

Tuck jumps
(knees to chest)
A1-20
A2-25
A3-30 ④

however, will allow you to retain agility and improve speed, acceleration and power in the legs and upper body.

At this level it is a good idea to familiarize yourself with correct
free-weight lifting techniques as well as machine-based equipment.

Once you have progressed safely through the transition goals, the following is a suggested programme at an advanced level:

Weeks 1-4

Exercises	Sets	Repetitions
free-weight bench	4	12-15
seated rows	4	12-15
leg press	4	12-15
hamstring curls	4	12-15
shoulder press	4	12-15
crunches	4	20-30

Weeks 5-8

Exercises	Sets	Repetitions
dead lifts	3-5	5-9
cleans	2-3	5
bench press	3-5	5-9
bent-over rows	3-5	5-9
shoulder press	3-5	5-9
crunches	4-6	20-40

Weeks 8-12

Optional: Specifically for muscle endurance development

Exercise	Strength & Power		Muscle Endurance	
	Sets	Repetitions	Sets	Repetitions
dead lifts	2-4	3-5	—	—
cleans	2-4	3-5	4-6	20
leg press	2-4	3-5	4-6	40
leg curls	2-4	3-5	4-6	20-40
bench press	2-4	3-5	4-6	40
seated rows/ bent-over rows	2-4	3-5	4-6	40
shoulder press	2-4	3-5	4-6	20
crunches	4-6	40	4-6	40

Developing speed and acceleration

Sprint drills, as discussed in the entry-level section, remain the basis of developing speed and acceleration. Having attained considerably greater strength levels through an extended strength-training programme, you can now take advantage of plyometrics. Chapter 7 details a number of drills appropriate to football (use the programme for advanced acceleration).

It's really important that you begin plyometric training only once you are completely warm by first doing a longish aerobic component and stretch (i.e. a 10-15 minute run then full stretch).

A speed and acceleration session would look as follows:

Component	Time (min)	Repetitions	Sets	Notes
warm-up	10-15	—	—	light aerobic jog/cycle/step at 60% of MHR
stretching	15	3 times on each side of the body		hold a moderate stretch for 15-20 sec in each repetition and repeat. Emphasize legs, calf and back
plyometrics	20	8-10 per set	4-6	keep the levels low to begin with and gradually build
sprint drills	20-30	6-8 per set	3-6	number of sets depends on distances run. Drills require 100% effort with walk back to the start as you rest between reps; 5-min rest (stretching) between sets
warm-down	5	—	—	light jog/cycle, etc. at 60% MHR
stretching	10	as before		as above

> The type of training activity is important. Remember, variety really is the spice of training life!

RUGBY

Rugby is played under two codes: Rugby League and the more widely played Rugby Union (both games consisting of two 40-minute halves). With 15 players in a Union team, you will always find a position to suit you regardless of your physical build or height. Every team requires fast, elusive backs whose speed is more important than their height, and other players tall enough to win the ball in line-outs. This huge variation in size is most often seen in Rugby Union due to the variety of game-play situations such as line-outs, scrums and loose play. In Rugby League players are generally all quite powerfully built as the game is (if we may say so without upsetting too many League players) more like a battering-ram. This chapter deals primarily with Rugby Union.

GENERAL CHARACTERISTICS OF THE RUGBY PLAYER

If you want to be a valuable team member you will need:

- a high level of skill with both your hands and feet
- a tough mental and physical approach.

Rugby is a difficult, challenging and hugely satisfying sport, but is way ahead of the field for regular knocks and the odd bump and cut! The game can be very demanding, especially if you play in the forwards. These players are almost continuously involved in wrestling for the ball – a practice known as 'rucking' or 'mauling'. There is a large element of contact, falling to the ground, having to pick yourself up time after time and sprinting to the next section of play to make a tackle. If you play in the backs, you will need to be as fast as possible with good off-the-mark acceleration. Backs are normally slightly smaller in stature – but there are some huge backs out there!

Basic physical requirements

Rugby is a complicated sport to prepare for and requires a diverse range of abilities. The physical requirements on the pitch are:

- strength
- acceleration
- power.

- aerobic stamina
- flexibility

How fit do I need to be to play?

Very fit, at all levels! A pick-up game with friends or on the odd Saturday may leave you quite stiff for a week! Rugby is a perfect example of the adage 'Be fit to play – don't play to get fit'. Both Rugby League and Union can be described as multiple-sprint sports. That is, regardless of your playing position you need to be able to work for periods of 10-50 seconds with rest periods lasting only 5-15 seconds for the whole game. How hard you work depends on the position you play; the backs tend to get slightly more rest than the forwards and are involved in play for slightly shorter periods. This disparity is less common in League than in Union.

Strength and muscle endurance

Your muscles must have the ability to keep contracting many thousands, if not tens of thousands, of times during a game. Strength is vital for developing acceleration and speed as well as for coping with constant tackling and mauling. It is no over-exaggeration to say that every muscle in the body is used in the game, either voluntarily or to support the joints as they are put under the multi-directional stresses associated with running angles, taking tackles and diving for tries.

Aerobic stamina

You will also need above-average aerobic stamina: the ability to keep on running is often the deciding factor between winning and losing. Aerobic stamina also improves short-sprinting ability.

Flexibility

Flexibility is often neglected by players and can be below average. So it is particularly important that you devote time and effort to it in your training.

Is injury inevitable?

Although the game involves heavy contact, especially in the forwards, close attention to physical preparation will lessen the likelihood of anything more than a few knocks and bumps, painful as they can be!

THE PLAYING YEAR

The season usually runs between September and May in Rugby Union, and November and May in Rugby League. However, it is quite possible to play virtually all year round, or to play a short season which encompasses just 1 of the several cup- and league-type competitions. All players should expect to be fitness training 3-5 days a week.

EQUIPMENT

The mouth guard (gum shield)

The right equipment is a must to ensure safety in play, and the most important piece is a mouth guard. Cheap ones are not good enough. Visit a dentist who understands the requirements of a contact sport and he or she will tailor a guard to suit you. The guard must be strong enough to withstand a considerable blow yet allow you to talk and breathe freely.

Boots

Buy a pair of boots you feel comfortable in. There are 3 different cuts of rugby boot:

1. A high cut which gives good ankle support and protection and is often favoured by props, hookers and locks.

2. A mid-cut, giving good protection and support while allowing greater bend at the ankle and a freer movement. This is worn by flankers and the number 8.

3. A low cut which gives minimal support and ankle protection but allows for the freest movement. This is worn by the backs from numbers 9 to 15, and quite often by the forwards who want to be backs!

Clothing

You need some strong training shorts, tops and wet-weather gear, all designed specifically for the game.

Kicking tee

Additionally, if you are a good place kicker, you will want your own kicking tee for practising this specific and delicate skill, as well as for use in the game.

ENTRY-LEVEL PROGRAMME

Rugby requires a good general level of fitness, particularly aerobic stamina and strength. You must begin by developing these 2 areas before moving on to more position-specific work.

Aerobic conditioning: the forwards

Excellent leg power and exceptional upper-body strength are required for all forward positions. Forwards should concentrate on developing a good aerobic level. Forwards tend to be heavy, muscular builds, and as such they have to work harder to move around the pitch. If some of that weight is excess fat, regular aerobic exercise and a healthy, low-fat diet will successfully reduce that fat and develop good aerobic stamina.

As heavily built players, forwards should be mindful of the extra stress placed on joints, in particular knees, back, hips and ankles. Running is an important part of training but you should include high- and low-impact training when you start out and concentrate on running training as you become stronger and the playing season draws near.

High-impact training involves activities such as running, jumping and sharp turning which put more stress on joints than low-impact activities such as rowing, walking, swimming, cycling or using the step machine, in which the body weight is supported and the impact on the joints is less. Both modes of training have benefits, although high-impact training is generally tailored more to a particular sport.

Begin by jogging slowly on soft, grassy surfaces. Save your heavy work for the step machine, rowing machine, etc. Vary the intensity and slowly build the duration of your training. We suggest this initial 6-week aerobic programme, but remember to find modes of training that suit you yet allow you to keep up the correct duration and intensity.

Week	Mode	Time (min)	Frequency per week	Intensity	Notes
1	mix cycling/ rowing/ stepping	20	3	50-60% MHR	get used to the time required
2	as above	25-35	3-4	60-70% MHR	as above
3	add 20-min jog	up to 40	4	60-70% MHR	begin running, build from 20-40 min
4	as above	as above	4	70-75% MHR	as above
5	try to run 2 × week	40-50	4-5	80-85% MHR	mix heavy sessions with easier ones such as cycling
6	as above running 3 × week	as above	4-5	80-85% MHR	as above

Aerobic conditioning: the backs

Although muscular, back players are usually quite lean. As a back you should find continuous running relatively easy and it is unlikely you will suffer joint-stress problems as some forwards do unless you are already predisposed to injury. You should follow the same aerobic programme as suggested for the forwards, but try to introduce running earlier in the programme, say in weeks 1-2.

Working on strength: resistance training

This is the part that most players prefer. To make good, consistent gains you should be lifting weights at least 3 times a week. Use a high-weight, low-repetition programme as this will rapidly improve your general strength (see Chapter 5 for recommended exercises). If you are an experienced lifter, or once you have completed the initial 4- to 6-week programme, it is advisable to move from machine-based weight routines to include some simple free-weight exercises.

Pre-season training

Now that you've completed a solid 8-12 weeks of groundwork you should look to begin more specific work. This means that you will need to consider the requirements of your team position in a little more detail.

Pre-season training should take you 4-6 weeks depending on how much foundation, strength and aerobic work you have put in. The better the base, the less time it will take you to achieve good specific fitness. Pre-season is also a time when most clubs begin club training. This means that you will be involved in a combination of skills training and fitness training. If your club runs a fitness-training session you should work out if it's a speed session, aerobic session or some other type, and then adjust your schedule accordingly.

All Rugby League positions should complete the suggested work for group 3.

Group 1: the props

As you are big players it is particularly important for you to establish good running fitness. Your muscular stature means that you must be aware of any joint discomfort; if any occurs and persists over a 2-week period, seek medical attention and reduce the amount of running you do. You'll find the running a challenge for sure, but stick with it!

Week	Mode	Time (min)	Frequency per week	Intensity	Notes
1	running/rowing	20	3	85% MHR	keep a constant high pace
2	running/rowing	30-40	3	90% MHR	work at 90% for 2 min and then drop the pace for 3 min to 40%
3	running/rowing /cycling	30	3	as above	as above
4	swim/step/cycle	40	3	85% MHR	as for week 1
5	running	40	3	interval running at 90% MHR	as for week 2
6	as for week 5	40	3	as above	as for week 2

Group 2: the locks

As tall players you will need a combination of running pace, jumping ability and strength. Incorporate some simple, plyometric jump-training exercises. However, still continue your upper-body strength work and improve your running pace.

Week	Mode	Time (min)	Frequency per week	Intensity	Notes
1	plyometrics		1	100% effort	see entry-level jump programme in Chapter 7
	upper-body strength		2		as per entry level
	2 × wk running	20	2	85% MHR	continuous running at constant pace
2	plyometrics		1	100% effort	see entry-level jump programme in Chapter 7
	upper-body strength		2		as per entry level
	2 × wk running	30-40	2	85% MHR	continuous running at constant pace
3	plyometrics		1	100% effort	see entry-level jump programme in Chapter 7
	upper-body strength		2		as per entry level
	interval running	30-40	2	90% MHR	begin interval running 2 min at 90% MHR; follow by 3 min at 60% MHR; complete 3 rotations of this then jog for 5 min at 50%; complete this circuit 2-3 times
4	as above	as above	1:2:2	as above	as above
5	run/cycle/step	as above	1:2:2	as above	as above
6	as for week 3	as above	1:2:2	as above	as above

Group 3: the flankers, number 8, hooker and scrum half

Week	Mode	Time (min)	Frequency per week	Intensity	Notes
1	upper-body strength		1-2		as for your foundation strength training
	plyometrics		1	100%	follow the entry-level acceleration programme in Chapter 7
	continuous running	30	2	85%	keep a constant pace, but try to incorporate some slight hills
2	as above, but begin interval running	running time 30-40		running intervals up to 90% MHR	running intervals of 1 min as fast as possible followed by 1 min at 50% MHR; complete 6 of these rotations then jog for 5 min; complete 3 circuits of this
3	as above, except cycle, step or run for interval work	as above		as above	as above
4	replace interval running with running drills (see overleaf)	see notes		as above	complete running drill 1; complete 6 reps; rest, stretching for 2 min between sets; complete 2 sets; all other training remains as is
5	incorporate running drill 2	see notes		as above	complete 1 set of reps for both drill 1 and drill 2; rest for 2 min between each set
6	as above	see notes		as above	complete 2 sets of drill 1 and 1 set of drill 2

Running drills for pre-season training

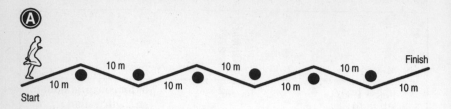

1. Sprint to the 1st marker. Fall onto the marker as if it were a loose ball in play. Feed the ball back, get up and sprint to the next marker.
2. Continue for all the markers/balls then jog half-way back and walk half-way back to the start. This is one repetition.

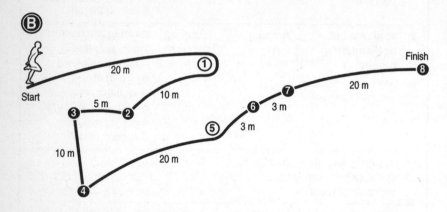

1. As above, except run around markers 1 and 5 and fall on markers 2, 3, 4, 6, 7, 8.
2. Continue for all the markers/balls then jog half-way back and walk half-way back to the start. This is one repetition.

If you are a scrum half you are probably wondering why you should be training with the back-row boys. This is because part of your game is more like a forward than a back. Your running pattern is more similar to that of a flanker than an inside centre. You may not do as much tackling as your colleagues in this training group but you certainly do as much running.

Groups 4 and 5: the centres, wings and full backs
Base, pre-season programmes for these groups are similar.

Week	Mode	Time (min)	Frequency per week	Intensity	Notes
1	upper-body strength/size		2	100% effort	follow the strength/size routine suggested in Chapter 5
	plyometrics		1	100% effort	follow the entry-level acceleration programme in Chapter 7
	running	30	2	85% MHR	use plenty of variation in terrain
2	as above; replace continuous running with interval running	see notes	2:1:2		complete 6 reps of each of the following distances: 10 m, 30 m, 60 m; walk-back recovery after each rep; 5 min stretching recovery between each set
3	as above and see notes	see notes	2:1:2	see notes	complete level 1 of your position-specific running drills (see overleaf); all other training remains the same
4	as above	as above	2:1:2	see notes	complete level 2 of your position-specific running drills
5	as above	as above	2:1:2	see notes	complete level 3 of your position-specific running drills
6	as above	as above	2:1:2	see notes	as above

The variations in these 2 groups' requirements are in distances run, rest intervals and running patterns. Overleaf are specialized running drills that give each position its specific training effect.

Running drills for fly half, inside centre and outside centre

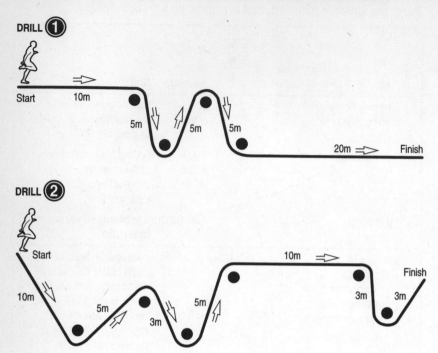

Sprint around each of the markers. Ensure you go around the marker (use a pole flag if possible) not over it. Concentrate on achieving a powerful, sharp side step at each marker.

Level	Notes
Level 1, week 3	complete 6 repetitions per set; walk back between each sprint; complete 3 sets and rest, stretching for 5 min between sets; use drill 1 only
Level 2, week 4	complete 8 repetitions per set; complete 1 set of drill 1 and 1 set of drill 2; recovery as for week 3
Level 3, weeks 5 & 6	complete 6 repetitions per set; complete 2 sets of drill 1 and 2 sets of drill 2; recovery as for week 3

Running drills for wings and full backs

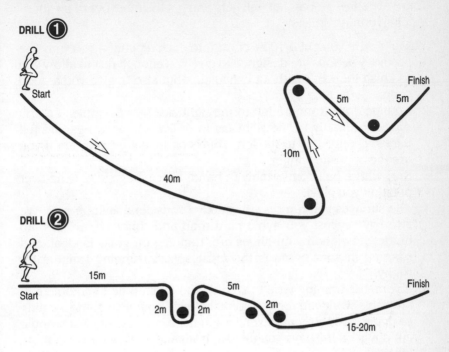

Level	Notes
Level 1, week 3	complete 4 repetitions per set; jog and half walk-back recovery; complete 3 sets of drill 1 with 5 min stretching rest between sets
Level 2, week 4	complete 2 sets of drill 1 and 2 sets of drill 2; complete 5 repetitions per set; recovery as for week 3
Level 3, weeks 5 & 6	complete 6 repetitions per set; complete 3 sets of each drill; recovery as for week 3

Getting the most out of position-specific training

There are a few points that will help you get the most out of position-specific running drills:

1. Make sure you put a 100% effort into each repetition you run. The recovery periods are designed to give you enough rest to allow you to finish the work without exhaustion but also to give you a good training effect.
2. Change drills from the left to the right side. For example, if a drill moves primarily to the right (as in drill 2 for the wings and full backs) change this to the left. This is particularly important if you are the opposite winger.
3. Run with a ball comfortably in hand, alternating sides (whatever position you play).
4. The surfaces you run on also make a considerable difference. We strongly suggest you avoid hard road and concrete surfaces, no matter how good your shoes are. Running on grass is ideal, and running in your boots is the most specific running training for rugby.
5. Plyometric training won't take you too much time to complete. If after this work you feel reasonably fresh, complete some running or upper-body strength exercises in the same session. This should cut down on the days you need to train and make your week more efficient.
6. Always complete plyometrics first if you are going to do more than one type of training in a session. It is important to be fresh and rested before plyometric training if you are to get the most out of it.

Here are some suggested programmes for pre-season training:

Pre-season training week: 1 session per day	
Mon	running or other aerobic or intervals
Tues	plyometrics
Wed	running or other aerobic or intervals
Thurs	strength (upper body)
Fri	rest
Sat	strength (upper body)
Sun	rest

Pre-season training week: some double sessions	
Mon	plyometrics and upper-body strength
Tues	running or other aerobic or intervals
Wed	plyometrics and upper-body strength
Thurs	running or other aerobic or intervals
Fri	rest
Sat	optional training day or rest
Sun	rest

TRANSITION GOALS

If you have started with the entry-level programme, these transition goals will indicate how your training has been progressing and whether you are ready to go on to the advanced training schedule:

1. You should possess a good-quality mouth guard.
2. You must have good-quality boots and trainers, both in good repair.
3. You should be able to run reasonably comfortably at 85% of your MHR for 40 minutes.
4. You should be able to complete all the position-specific training drills suggested for your position.
5. You must be free of injury. This includes minor muscle strains.
6. Your diet should include at least 2 litres of water a day (pure water, not that drunk in tea, coffee, etc.) and at least 60% good-quality carbohydrate.
7. You must have completed a minimum of 6 weeks' consistent resistance (weight) training. The ideal is to have achieved a 30% improvement in the weight/resistance you are lifting. This is a minimum level and many of you will exceed this, but some may be below the level.
8. If you began at entry level, you must have completed at least 80% of the programme. If you have done this, then goals 3, 4 and 7 should be a breeze!

ADVANCED-LEVEL TRAINING

At this level you probably have been playing the game for a couple of seasons and have been training for at least 2 years. You should be able to satisfy all the transition goals. Take some time to read through the entry-level programme to familiarize yourself with the general approach and terminology as we'll be getting straight down to business from here on.

Laying your foundations – an excellent aerobic level

Without significantly beefing up your aerobic level (VO_2) you will struggle to complete the pre-season position-specific work; you'll also find that, having successfully completed level 1 of this work, you will be pushed to keep on improving. You simply must get the work done! The following aerobic programme should be completed by all players:

Week	Mode	Time (min)	Frequency per week	Intensity	Notes
1	run or cycle	40	4	70%	keep to flat terrain; soft running surfaces
2	run, swim, row, step or cycle	45	5	80-85%	rotate through your preferred modes
3	as above	60	4	75-80%	lower the intensity slightly
4	run	60	5	80-85%	work for 5 min at 85% then drop to 80% for 5 min; repeat for 60 min
5	run	45	4	65-70%	a lighter week but still important in the overall plan
6	run	40	4	85%	complete these runs as fast as you can; only complete 2 sessions if you are not doing weeks 7 and 8
*7	As for week 3, but complete only 3 sessions				
*8	As for week 2, but complete only 2 sessions				

*Additional, optional weeks. Recommended if you can find the time

106

The strength base

You can never have enough strength for rugby. Greater power and acceleration (backed up by a good engine, i.e. your aerobic level) can be achieved only by increasing your strength. Working solely on power without first working on strength will yield only small improvements. Having said that, you do have to work on power and acceleration if you want to improve them – that is what pre-season training is designed for.

At this level, you will have done some consistent resistance training. After several weeks of training on a particular routine you will have noticed that achievements level off. This happens because, after a while, your nervous and muscular systems tend to become accustomed to the work more rapidly. The following programme, however, will encourage progress as you only have a few weeks on any one routine before moving on to another. This provides a training stimulus to the muscles, preventing the levelling-off effect (known as 'desensitization') to some degree. Please refer back to Chapter 5 for recommended exercises.

Week	Frequency per week	Repetitions / sets	Resistance	Notes
1	3	5-9 / 3-5	very high	develops good overall strength; there is only a moderate amount of increased bulk; players looking for greater mass should follow the repetitions and sets for weeks 7 and 8
2	3	5-9 / 3-5	very high	
3	3	5-9 / 3-5	very high	
4	3	40+ / 4-6	low-medium	increases local endurance in the muscle, crucial for continuous top-speed running and mauling
5	3	40+ / 4-6	low	
6	3	40+ / 4-6	low	
7	3	4-6 / 12-15	high	upper-body strength only, as above
8	3	4-6 / 12-15	high	

The pre-season frenzy

If you have completed the recommended foundation work on your strength and aerobic base, you will find the following work far more manageable and even enjoyable! You should feel very well prepared after this work.

Group 1: the props

Week	Mode	Time (min)	Frequency per week	Intensity	Notes
1	strength		2	100%	as for weeks 7 and 8 of foundation training (see page 106)
	running	40	3	85-90%	1 × week intervals: 6 × 300 m, half walk-back, half jog-back recovery; 2 × week 40 min at top pace
2	as above	40		as above	as above, increase intervals to 8 × 300 m
3	as above	30-40	4	as above	2 × week intervals: 8 × 360 m and 4 × 200 m; recovery as for week 1; 30 min 2 × week as fast as possible
4	strength		4	as above	intervals: work at maximum for 2 min, then 1 min working very light; repeat for 30 min; run for the other 2 sessions, as for week 3
5	running, strength work			otherwise as for week 3	
6	as above; increase intervals to 8 × 300 m and then 6 × 200 m				

Group 2: the locks

Week	Mode	Time (min)	Frequency per week	Intensity	Notes
1	upper-body strength	40	2	100%	upper-body strength as for weeks 7 and 8 of foundation training (see page 106)
	plyometrics	20	1	100%	follow the advanced-level jump programme in Chapter 7
	running	40	2	85%	continuous running, varied terrain
2	as above except for running		2	interval training	6 × 400 m at 90% MHR, 200-m half jog and half walk recovery, then complete 6 × 300 m, recovery as above
3	as above	as above		increase repetitions	increase repetitions to 2 sets of 6 × 300 m and 1 set of 6 × 400 m
4	as above	as above		vary interval distances	3 sets of 6 repetitions over 40 m and 3 sets of 6 repetitions over 10 m; complete this 1 × week and week 3 work 1 × week
5		as above	as above	as above	as above
6		as above	as above	as above	as above

You are having to complete 5 sessions a week in the final 6 weeks to the start of the season, so it is vital that you first have a good strength, aerobic and flexibility base. You'll find it particularly taxing to undertake this level of work without good basic preparation. Equally, you'll improve rapidly in the period if you've been vigilant in the previous 6-8 weeks.

Hillsborough College

Learning Resource Centre
Telephone: 0114 2602254

Group 3: the flankers, number 8, hooker and scrum half

Week	Mode	Time (min)	Frequency per week	Intensity	Notes
1	upper-body strength	30	2	100%	complete bench press, seated rows, military press and abdominal crunches; use the strength-training schedule in Chapter 5
	plyometrics	20	1	100%	follow the advanced-level acceleration programme in Chapter 7
	interval running	40	2	90%+	6 × 300 m half jog and half walk-back recovery, then 6 × 200 m, recovery as above
2	as above for strength and plyometrics	as above		vary interval running	complete 1 × 6 reps of the sprint drills 1 and 2 opposite, then complete 1 set of 6 repetitions of 300 m; all recoveries as above
3	as above	as above		see notes	2 × 6 reps drill 1, 3-min rest between sets; 2 × 6 reps drill 2, rest as above
4	as above	as above		as above	6 × 200 m; 2 × 6 reps drill 1; 2 × 6 reps drill 2; rest and recovery as above
5	as above	as above		as above	as above
6	as above	as above		as above	3 × 6 reps drill 1; 2 × 6 reps drill 2; rest and recovery as above

Speed endurance drills

DRILL ①

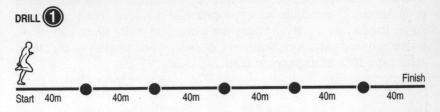

Sprint from the start to mark 1. At mark 1 fall on a ball and feed it back as you would in the game. Alternatively, do one press-up. Get up as quickly as possible and sprint as hard as possible to mark 2. Again, fall to the ground, etc. Repeat to mark 6. Jog back immediately to mark 3 and then walk to the start. This is one repetition.

DRILL ②

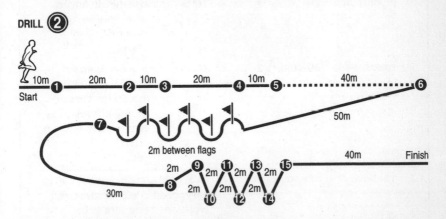

Sprint between marks 1-5 as for drill 1. Sprint backwards between marks 5-6. At mark 6 complete 30 press-ups. Sprint to, and then in and out of the flags. You should ensure you do not touch any flag. At mark 7 complete 30 burpees (see page 137). At mark 8 complete 14-m lateral movements with only a 2- to 5-m forward movement. At each mark touch the ground with the outside hand. Bend low and aim for a powerful lateral push/drive away from the mark. Sprint to the finish. This is one repetition.

Remember: it is *vital* that you work as hard as you can in all phases of the drill – there must be no half-paced running! Recovery as for drill 1.

Groups 4 and 5: the centres, wings and full backs

Use the position-specific drills already described in the entry-level programme. These drills are appropriate at this level, but you should go a little further. Analyse your own game and make slight variations to the running patterns (directions, distances and angles) so that they reflect the style of rugby your team is playing.

Week	Mode	Time (min)	Frequency per week	Intensity	Notes
1	strength	40	2	100%	follow strength/bulk routine, upper body only
	plyometrics	20	1	100%	use the advanced-level acceleration programme in Chapter 7
	speed	30–40	2	100%	1 × 6 reps 40 m, 1 × 6 reps 20 m, 1 × 6 reps 15 m; walk-back recovery between reps; 5 min stretching between sets
2	as above	as above	as above	as above, vary speed work; see notes	2 × 6 reps over 40 m, 2 × 6 reps for drills 1 and 2 for your position
3	as above	as above	as above	as above	as above
4	as above	as above	as above	as above	3 × 6 reps of drill 1, 4 × 6 reps of drill 2; walk-back recovery between reps and 5 min (stretching) between sets; you need a full recovery between sets
5	as above	as above	as above	as above	as above
6	as above	as above	as above	as above	as above

Remember, real gains depend on the quality of your work. A move up to advanced level should be reflected in how much *effort* you put into training. More time spent training is not necessarily better! Depending on the time you have available, you can decide whether to follow a single or double daily workout schedule. Examples of these are given in the entry-level section on pages 104-5.

HOCKEY

Hockey, like rugby, is a multiple-sprint team sport. It is typified by brief bursts of high-intense exercise (the sprint) in between periods of lower-intensity recovery (walking or jogging). The game has two 35-minute halves, with a 5- to 10-minute break. Overall it is fast in pace, but the majority of fast bursts last only between half a second and 2 seconds, with only 5% lasting longer than 7 seconds. Such brief sprints highlight the importance of *acceleration*.

THE TEAM

A team, which can play in varied formations, comprises 11 players and is made up of the following positions:

- goalkeeper
- defenders
- midfield players
- forwards.

Playing hockey well requires a wide repertoire of skills, both physical and technical, and you need to focus on all these in your training. Most of you who play hockey regularly with a club will probably be doing skill and technical training. But you must also undertake fitness training.

ENERGY DEMANDS

First and foremost you need to be fit for hockey. You need:

- a reasonable level of fitness
- stamina
- acceleration
- good aerobic fitness.

A lot of the work in hockey is done 'off the ball' – marking, getting into position, chasing. This allows you to recover from the energy-intensive times when you are dribbling the ball in a bent-over position. Dribbling with the ball increases both heart rate (up to 23 bpm) and energy expenditure to approximately 15% more than normal running with a stick at the same speed. Clearly, you would be exhausted if you played the whole game in that position.

How strenuous is it?

On average, you can expect to cover 5-8 km in a full game. During this time, you would be exercising at about 78% of your maximum aerobic capacity (see Chapter 2 for information on how to measure your maximum aerobic capacity). This is quite tough. Depending on the level you play at – a fun social game or a good standard of club hockey – you would probably burn 9-15 kilocalories per minute during the game. Games tend to be much faster, and therefore you use more calories, on the newer synthetic surfaces. At the very top levels you play even faster and can burn up to 17 kilocalories per minute – 1240 kilocalories in 1 game.

Which muscles do you use most?

- As a running sport, hockey primarily uses the muscles in the front and back of the thigh, the backside and the calves.
- The shoulder muscles are probably the next most used as they initiate the swing and carry the stick while you are running.
- The biceps and triceps at the front and back of the upper arm do a certain amount of work in controlling the ball, particularly while you are dribbling.
- The muscles and joints of the lower back come under a lot of stress and strain in hockey as the bent-over position when dribbling the ball is not the most natural or comfortable of positions to run in. You can avoid unnecessary back strain by incorporating back-strengthening and flexibility exercises into your training programme.

PLAYER PROFILE

There is no ideal physique as the skill aspect of the game overrides pure physical attributes. If you are good technically and tactically, your height and size don't really matter. However, the best players tend to have a fairly muscular body shape which helps when tackling or hitting two-handed. This is the case for both men and women.

Body fat

Women players tend to have the same amount of body fat as the average, relatively non-active person. Levels average at 22-25% at county level. However, at the highest levels of play and around the time of peak fitness at international competitions body-fat levels in women players are reduced to 16-26% – a huge range. Low body fat, therefore, is not essential to succeed as a female hockey player. Men playing at county or good club level have relatively low amounts of body fat: about 10-12%.

Aerobic capacity

For women at international level, and below, the required aerobic capacity is similar to that for lacrosse players, lower than that for runners and orienteers, and higher than that for netball players. The difference between competitive standards is relatively small, with English national squad players having a VO_2 max of about 46 ml/kg/min and county players levels of about 41 ml/kg/min. This would be a little higher at peak time in the playing season. Men would expect to have VO_2 max levels of 48-65 ml/kg/min. Naturally, these ranges differ according to the standard of the player and team, and the position in the team.

EQUIPMENT

Shoes

Having the correct shoes is as important in hockey as in any sport. You will probably need 2 pairs of shoes: one for grass and the other for artificial turf. You can choose from 2 types for the grass-pitch games (aim for a good comfortable fit with good heel cushioning):

1. The shoe-like boot that goes further up your ankle and gives more support.
2. Some hockey players choose to wear *football b*oots, which are broadly similar but with a harder toe.

> Ensure you are at your fittest at that time of the year when your club has its most important games.

Special artificial turf shoes are available, but a good pair of running trainers with a decent grip is perfectly adequate.

Stick and shin pads

The crook of the stick has become smaller in recent years to allow better ball control. If you prefer, however, go for a bigger head. Also, the majority of sticks are no longer made of wood, but of aluminium or Kevlar, both of which make the stick more rigid and allow you to hit the ball further (because less energy is lost in vibrations within the stick when you hit the ball). However, if you feel more comfortable with a wooden stick, stay with it as you will not play your best if your equipment does not feel right. Some strong shin pads are also essential, but the rest of the clothing is entirely up to you and the team you play with.

THE PLAYING YEAR

Hockey is a seasonal game played mostly over the winter months from September to April. Most clubs at all levels play weekly matches. It is difficult to define a peak in this long season as this depends on the level of the club. Most clubs, no matter what division, will have a mixture of league or cup matches and 'friendly' matches.

ENTRY-LEVEL TRAINING

If you are getting back into hockey after several years off, or if you are taking it up as a new sport, your first goals will be to get yourself aerobically fit enough to last the whole game. Then, you can introduce more specific acceleration and speed training. Naturally, skill training will be important. Coping with the weekly knocks and bruises may also take some getting used to! Beyond this, it is a matter of time, personal goals and individual skill level as to how far you progress.

- If you prefer to play at a more social and recreational level, and not necessarily every week, follow the entry-level training programme.
- If you are already playing regularly, are reasonably fit, want to progress to a better team or level, or feel that your game could be improved, then follow the advanced training programme.

Hockey is very demanding on your aerobic system so you must develop great stamina. Your training should include the running patterns of the sport: running forwards, backwards and sideways. About 30-40% of play (including running and tackling) involves a bent-over stance, so include this in your training as the season draws near.

Weeks 1-4

For the first 4 weeks concentrate on non-specific, continuous, aerobic training. This means that you should rest your legs and use mostly non-weight-bearing activities to build your aerobic load. This is especially useful if you are recovering from the previous season's rigours or an injury.

Week	Mode	Duration (min)	Intensity	Frequency per week
1	cycle, swim or step machine	20-30	50-60% MHR	2
2	run, cycle, aerobic classes, swim	40-45	60-70% MHR	3
3	as above	40-50	65-75% MHR	3-4
4	as above	40-50	75-85% MHR	3-4

Weeks 5-6

Now you should do the following interval training. This training will put you in good shape for the final 4-6 weeks before you begin playing:

Week	Mode	Duration (min)	Frequency per week	Details
5	run or step machine	30-40	3	5 min at 50% MHR; 1 min at 85-90% of MHR (or 400 m) then 2 min at 50% of MHR (or 200 m); complete this cycle 6 times then jog for 5 min at 40% MHR
6	run	40-50	3	as above, except work for 1 min 30 sec at 85-90% and rest for 3 min at 50% MHR

What kind of running?
You need to emphasize the short, sharp intervals you run. Try to mirror how you run in a game; each distance may be as short as in your game, but the total training time must equal the duration of a game.
The 3 main running exercises are:

- multi-directional running (running with quick changes in direction)
- speed off the mark (acceleration from standing)
- short bursts of very high-intensity running (running with quick pace changes or acceleration).

It is very important to remember to maintain the aerobic base you have developed to date. Do this by completing 1 running session and 1 other session of either swimming, rowing machine, step machine or cycling. These sessions should last 40 minutes.

Weeks 7-12: speed and anaerobic threshold development

You should complete 2 other speed/speed-endurance sessions. They should be as follows:

Week	Duration (min)	Details
7	40-45	drill A (overleaf) drill B (overleaf) drill C (overleaf)
8	40-50	repeat the drills as above, dribbling a ball for half the sets (except when you are running backwards); complete 5 press-ups for every error
9	45-50	as above except halve all repetitions per set for each exercise (A-C) and add drill D (overleaf)
10	45-50	complete as for week 9
11	45-50	complete as for week 9 but now try to increase the repetitions per set back up to those in week 7
12	45-50	add in the penalty press-ups for any mistakes

Drills for speed and anaerobic threshold development

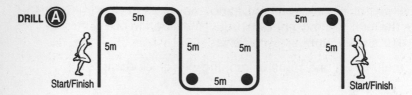

DRILL Ⓐ

Sprint through the drill. Rest for 15 seconds at the finish, then go back the other way. Complete 8 repetitions per set. Complete 2 sets. Rest 5 min between sets. Complete half the sets dribbling a ball.

DRILL Ⓑ

Sprint over 20-40 m. Carry your stick for all sprints. Complete 6 repetitions in a set. Walk back to the start as recovery between repetitions. Rest for 3 min between sets. Complete 2 sets.

DRILL Ⓒ

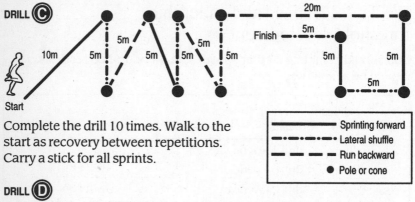

Complete the drill 10 times. Walk to the start as recovery between repetitions. Carry a stick for all sprints.

————	Sprinting forward
—·—·—·—	Lateral shuffle
— — — —	Run backward
●	Pole or cone

DRILL Ⓓ

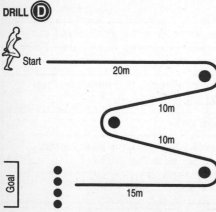

Perform drills A-C, halving the repetitions throughout. Then add the following drill. Sprint the drill with your stick in hand. When reaching the balls shoot each of them into the goal. The goal should be 5-15 m away. Replace the balls and walk to the start. Complete 8-10 repetitions.

Strength training

Don't forget that strength does not always mean a big increase in size; nor does it lead to a decrease in speed or flexibility. It can enhance them both! Strength is of great benefit to you but running ability (stamina) is the most important skill. With this in mind, you need only complete 2 weight-training sessions per week, in addition to your aerobic training.

When should you weight train?

Do your weight training on alternate days for no more that 40 minutes per session. Complete the following programme over the full 10-12 weeks of your overall preparation period. This is what your training week looks like:

Mon	Tues	Wed	Thurs	Fri	Sat	Sun
aerobic	weights	aerobic	weights	aerobic	rest	aerobic

Aerobic days include speed/speed endurance in weeks 5-10 and week 12 depending on the overall length of your build-up.

Weight-training exercises

Exercise	Sets(*1)	Repetitions	Loads(*2)
half squat or leg press (*3)	2-4	9-11	80-100%
leg curls (*3)	3-5	10-12	80-100%
bench press	2-4	9-11	80-100%
lateral pull downs	2-4	9-11	80-100%
shoulder press	3-5	10-12	80-100%
abdominal crunches	4	20-40	Body weight only

*1 Include a warm-up set of 10-15 repetitions at 50% effort.
*2 Loads should increase from 70% to 80% of your maximum in weeks 1-3; and to maximum effort (failure) in week 4 onwards.
*3 Progress from using both legs to complete these exercises to using 1 leg. The weight should be decreased when this transition occurs.

Flexibility

In the section on cycling (page 204) there are 2 great exercises in the advanced-level programme designed to counteract the rounded-shoulder syndrome often seen in riders. This same problem can occur in hockey players as they too spend a considerable amount of time in a stooped stance. Complete those exercises and also the ones below.

Quadriceps stretch

Lean back at the hips. The stretch should be felt in the thigh of the leg on the box. The angle of this leg is no less than 45 degrees and can be greater.

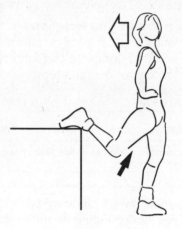

Combined groin and hip flexor stretch

Again, keep the back (stretched) leg at a good angle, no less than 45 degrees, and the upper body well back. Now turn sideways, pivoting on the front foot, with the other leg straight out to the side. The stretch sensation will change in the inner thigh/groin area.

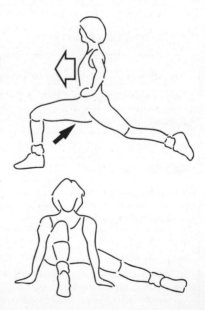

TRANSITION GOALS

You must be able to agree with the following before you contemplate moving on to advanced training:

1. You have completed 40 minutes of continuous aerobic work at 80% of MHR, 3–4 times a week over 3 weeks.
2. You have completed all of weeks 7-12 training at entry level.
3. You have completed a minimum of 8 weeks' uninterrupted weight training for strength.
4. You have no injuries that interfere in any way with your training.
5. You have good training equipment (especially shoes) in good repair.
6. Your diet includes at least 70% complex carbohydrate on a regular basis and you consume at least 1 litre of water a day.

ADVANCED-LEVEL TRAINING

At top level hockey is a fast, non-stop running game. Rarely do players have the opportunity to do anything less than jog to the next phase of play. You need excellent aerobic levels, explosiveness off the mark and the ability to hold an opponent off the ball with superior upper-body strength. If you are a midfield player you have the toughest job of linking backs and forwards. Your general stamina, especially your ability to work (run) at near maximum for the entire game, is always tested.

Have you met the requirements set out in the transition goals above? If so, you will have a good aerobic level but may need a 'top up' in some areas. If so, go back to the appropriate stage in the entry-level programme.

Aerobic capacity, speed endurance and acceleration

In addition to the work shown overleaf, complete at least 1 and preferably 2 × 30- to 40-minute, continuous aerobic sessions per week. Run for one session and do a mix of cycling, swimming, rowing and circuit-training classes for the other.

8-week pre-season programme – midfield players

Week	Frequency per week	Details
1	2	4 × 400 m sprints. Walk 200 m between repetitions as recovery; complete 4 per set; rest for 3 min between sets; complete 2 sets
2	2	as above but increase repetitions to 6 per set; increase sets to 3
3	3	4 × 200 m sprints; 3 sets of 6 repetitions per set; then complete 4 × 300 m. Again, 6 repetitions per set; complete 2 sets; all rests are as above
4	3	complete the drills outlined in week 7 of the entry-level programme; however, complete 8 repetitions per set; complete 2 sets each of drills A-C, of the entry-level programme (page 120)
5	3	as above, except complete two sets of 300 m sprints as per week 3 above, before completing the drills
6	3	as above
7	3	as for week 5, but now include drill D of the entry-level programme (page 120)
8	3	as above

8-week pre-season programme – forwards and backs

Week	Frequency per week	Details
1	2	complete drills A-D outlined in week 7 of the entry-level programme (page 120); complete 10 repetitions per set and 2 sets of each
2	3	as above
3	3	complete 2 sets of 6 repetition sprints over 20 m; walk to the start between reps and rest for 2 min between sets; now complete the work above (week 2)
4	2	complete the entry-level plyometric acceleration programme for weeks 3 and 4 (page 74); then complete drills A-D once only; complete 8 repetitions of each exercise
5	3	complete 1 session as week 4; then 2 sessions of week 3
6	3	complete 1 session of week 5, replacing the plyometric drills with those detailed for weeks 1 and 2 of the advanced acceleration programme (page 75); complete 2 sessions of week 1
7	3	as for week 6, plus 2 advanced plyometric sessions and 1 session as for week 1 above
8	2	as for week 3

Strength and power

You need upper-body strength to muscle your way past opponents and get into scoring positions. However, it is equally important to maintain your speed and speed endurance. So your programme needs to build strength without adding too much weight. Your leg strength is already likely to be well developed. As a forward or back, you will find that the plyometric exercises detailed above will help improve your acceleration and speed. If you have difficulty with these, increase your leg strength before progressing. Do this by adding the following exercises to your programme:

Extra exercises for leg strength
If you are a midfield player, speed endurance is all important. Your ability to run all match long is well developed through your aerobic/speed-endurance training. It is unlikely that, at this level, you will need additional leg strength. If you do, these exercises should be included in your upper-body strength programme.

Exercise	Sets	Reps	Loads
single-leg half squat	3	7-9	if you add these to your programme, you must stop any plyometric work;
single-leg curl	3	7-9	complete these exercises instead; complete 6 weeks of work before re-establishing plyometric work from week 4

Combined weekly training programme

Mon	aerobic (speed endurance) or speed
Tues	strength and continuous aerobic
Wed	aerobic (speed endurance) or speed
Thurs	strength
Fri	aerobic (speed endurance) or speed
Sat	rest
Sun	continuous aerobic

Upper-body development programme
Run this programme concurrently with your aerobic/speed training. You can even start your strength work 4 weeks earlier. This would make your strength programme 12 weeks long and your aerobic/speed training 8 weeks long. If you do this, you may wish to weight train on Monday, Wednesday and Friday for the first 4 weeks, then change to the weekly schedule suggested above.

There are 2 phases to the upper-body programme:

Weeks 1-4

Exercises	Sets	Reps	Loads
bench press	3-5	5-9	
lateral pull down	3-5	5-9	all to failure
shoulder press	3-5	5-9	
abdominal crunches	4	30-40	

Weeks 5-8 or 5-12

Exercise	Sets	Reps	Loads
pec fly	3-4	5-9	
bench press	3	7-9	
seated row	3-4	5-9	all to failure
lateral pull down	3	7-9	
shoulder press	3	7-9	
abdominal crunches	4	40-60	

Flexibility and additional training

Complete a thorough warm-up and warm-down before and after each session. The advanced programme is demanding, and to complete it successfully you must remain supple. Follow the stretches suggested in Chapter 6 and those additional stretches outlined in the entry-level section on page 122. You may also find useful the stretches and wrist-strengthening exercises detailed in the golf section (page 197).

BASKETBALL

Basketball is played all year round, both indoors and out. The season for professional indoor players lasts from October to April. Club basketball, frequently based at local leisure centres, also follows this seasonal pattern, with less of a following during the summer months as more of us move to the outdoor sports.

GENERAL CHARACTERISTICS OF THE BASKETBALL PLAYER

Basketball is a high-speed and high-intensity game requiring a great amount of skill. The following are very important:

- good aerobic fitness
- excellent co-ordination and skills
- good leg strength and power
- well-developed spatial awareness. Good basketball players appear not to look at the person they are passing the ball to, often passing it ahead of a running player!
- good communication with fellow team members to avoid collisions, often the cause of injuries.

BASKETBALL BASICS

The game is broken down into 4 × 15-minute (or 2 × 30-minute) play periods with a set break in between. Substitutions and fouls occur frequently and cause stoppages in the game, allowing the players a brief rest time. Competitive games can last 90 minutes. A team has 12 players, but only 5 are on the court at any one time and you may play for only 30-40 minutes of the whole game time. This does not imply that basketball is an 'easy' game. When on court you work hard, covering a fair amount of ground, sprinting up and down the court (the rests are well needed and well earned). The work-to-rest ratio in basketball averages at 1:1.7 – that is, for every 10 seconds of activity you have 17 seconds' break. This is enough time for the high-intensity energy systems to replenish their fuel stores.

ENERGY SYSTEMS

Any game that lasts over 20 minutes places a demand on your aerobic system. Just how much depends on the active and rest periods. Basketball requires a good aerobic capacity and excellent anaerobic power for acceleration and speed in covering the court. Also, the fitter you are the faster you will recover from the high-speed bursts and the more easily you will be able to repeat them time and time again without showing the effects of fatigue.

In a team sport such as basketball a lack of endurance becomes very evident in the latter part of the game when tactical mistakes are made or you just don't seem to be in the right place at the right time (and are very likely to be substituted). You will be playing at about 80-90% of your maximum heart rate – a strenuous 170 bpm – and burning up about 10-16 kilocalories per minute. In the average game (if you were on court for 30 minutes) you would expect to use up 480-640 kilocalories.

MUSCLES AND ACTIONS

As basketball is a running sport, the quadriceps, hamstrings and calf muscles will be carrying you at high speed around the court. The muscles on the inside and outside of the thigh also need to be strong and flexible to cope with the rapid changes in direction and frequent side-step running action. A lot of basketball players use a combination of strength training, plyometrics and jump training to achieve a good, explosive leg strength. Plyometric jumping is very popular and helps to improve the co-ordination of neuromuscular skills and muscle strength. That is, it trains your muscles to contract faster. It is a form of plyometrics that involves jumping down off benches or steps of varying heights (40 cm is the best) and springing upwards on landing.

BENEFITS AND RISKS

For those of you who are new to the game or have done little or no training, basketball is a good sport to improve your all-round fitness levels. The most noticeable improvements will be:

- an increased aerobic capacity
- leg tone
- strength.

However, it is best that you do some basic aerobic fitness training first as it is easy to get carried away on your first session and push yourself too hard. The resultant aches and pains can be very demoralizing, and you are at risk of injuring yourself.

The regular basketball player can maintain whatever aerobic fitness and strength he or she has but with little further improvement. These need to be worked on in training. The most common injuries in basketball are at the ankle and knee from sudden turns, and occasional lower-back pain from the jumping action. Good shoes and good preparation can help avoid these.

EQUIPMENT

The most important pieces of equipment in basketball are the shoes. To begin with, a good pair of indoor training shoes or running shoes is acceptable. If you play regularly, however, you need proper basketball shoes. The 'boot' design helps support and protect the ankle and the cushioning provides support in the correct places. Make sure the boots fit well and are comfortable.

PLAYER PROFILE

Height

There is no doubt that basketball players are taller than most other athletes (except, perhaps, high jumpers). Height tends to increase from amateur club level to professional and national teams. The average height of the English National League players is about 191 cm for males and 180 cm for females. In the USA, the average male height is

200 cm, and 185 cm for females. This is not to say that those of you with more average heights should shy away from basketball. Quite often the shorter player is much more agile around the court and can weave around and about the taller players very effectively.

Body-fat and training levels

Body-fat levels are low – the typical basketball player is lean and muscular (extra weight is a hindrance to good jumping). At league or national levels body fat is in the range of 10-14% for males and 12-18% for females. In terms of fitness, VO_2 max levels for male players range from 40-60 ml/kg/min at league or national level and those for females from 39-57 ml/kg/min. These are similar to the levels we see in most team or multiple-sprint sports. Basketball players, however, perform well on leg-power tests with females reaching over 40 cm and males over 50 cm in jump tests.

ENTRY-LEVEL TRAINING

These are the important fitness components for basketball:

- aerobic capacity
- muscle endurance, particularly in the legs
- good jumping ability.

Muscle tightness

At entry level you may find that your lower legs, thighs and (in some instances) your lower back become a little tight. This is usually short-lived and should only occur 2-3 days after a heavy playing or training session. You should seek medical advice if this occurs for longer periods. This tightness is a result of the jumping, the start-stop, and the turning involved. These movements place big loads on your muscles, more so than in many other sports.

Stretching

To counteract these periods of stiffness, and to ensure you remain in top condition, it is vital that you stretch regularly. In particular, you should work on the lower-leg calf muscles, the thigh muscles and those of your lower back (see Chapter 6).

Preparation programme: weeks 1-4

Week	Duration per session (min)	Frequency per week	Intensity % of MHR	Notes
1	20	2	60%	use a combination of jogging, stepping or cycling
2	30	2-3	75%	as above, but use at least 1 running session
3	30	3	75-80%	2 running sessions
4	30-40	3	75-80%	as for week 1

Having done the preparation programme you will notice that you now have a shorter recovery time between periods of high-intensity effort and those of relatively low intensity during the game, or when you are on the bench. This indicates that your aerobic capacity is improving.

Interval training: weeks 5-8

If you are still finding it hard work when you are playing flat out, you need to do a little interval training. Over the next 4 weeks, it is a good idea to include some interval work in your training, and we suggest the programme illustrated in the chart on the facing page.

Resistance training

The aerobic work done in weeks 1-8 is by far the most important for you, and this type of training should remain your first priority. If you have the time you may also wish to add some resistance training. Refer to Chapter 5 and complete the entry-level programme of exercises.

- Your upper-body exercises should be based on a programme for general strength. This involves sets of 3-5 and repetitions of 7-9.
- Concentrate on muscle endurance in your leg programme, using repetitions of 30-40 in each set you complete.
- If you include resistance training in your overall programme, do so on alternate days (such as Tuesday and Thursday). This may clash

Week	Duration per session (min)	Frequency per week	Intensity % of MHR	Mode	Notes
Interval training: weeks 5-8					
5	30-35	3 for continuous session; 2 for interval session	60% for continuous; 90% for intervals	cycle, step or jog for continuous; sprint for intervals	as for weeks 1-4 for continuous; intervals 1 min as fast as possible (consistent pace) then 2 min at 50%; complete 8-12 cycles of this work
6	as for week 5 above				
7	40	as for week 5	75% for continuous; 90% for intervals	as for week 5	intervals: 5 reps of 1 min on, 2 min off (full effort and 50% respectively); then 5-7 reps of 30 sec on, 15 sec off; complete 4 sets of this work
8	as for week 7 above				

with your planned aerobic sessions, but it's quite acceptable to complete both on the same day (but have a reasonable rest between each session).

TRANSITION GOALS

Before you consider moving on to the advanced training programme, or even starting at that point, ensure you can comfortably meet all of the following transition goals:

1. Continuous running for 35 minutes at 70-75% of your MHR.
2. Continuous biking or stepping for 50 minutes at 70-75% of your MHR.
3. You must have no injuries restricting your training.
4. Be stretching comfortably for 10-15 minutes in both the warm-up and cool-down periods.
5. Complete all of the recommended interval running.

6. Follow a diet in which complex carbohydrate makes up at least 50% of your total food intake.
7. Drink at least 6 glasses of water a day.
8. Own a good pair of basketball shoes or boots.

ADVANCED-LEVEL TRAINING

At this stage we assume you are playing at a high level, possibly training several times a week (or even daily) in basketball skills. Strength is a significant factor as your game becomes more competitive and faster. Strength is particularly important in the legs, where it is a prerequisite for the explosive power needed to play. If you are new to resistance training, complete the entry-level exercises suggested in Chapter 5. Move on to the advanced-level exercises once you are familiar with these.

Emphasis in weeks 1-8:

	Training emphasis	
Week	Lower body	Upper body
1	muscle endurance	strength
2	muscle endurance	strength
3	strength	
4	strength	strength
5	strength	muscle endurance
6	strength	muscle endurance
7	strength	muscle endurance
8	strength	muscle endurance

Leg power

The game at top level involves explosive court transitions, superb jumping and aggressive driving. These demanding athletic movements require exceptional leg power. The first 8 weeks of the advanced-level training programme have concentrated on increasing leg strength. This strength is necessary to ensure your plyometric work yields good, safe results.

Begin your advanced-level jumps and acceleration programme in week 6 of the first 8 weeks and continue to week 12 of your overall programme. At this point it is a personal decision whether you keep up this training. Games and practice sessions will be getting quite intense by now and will probably leave you with only 2-3 conditioning sessions per week. You must decide if they should emphasize your running, strength or leg-power work.

Aerobic and anaerobic training

At this level, you will have a fair degree of aerobic condition. The objective is to develop your ability to run, fast, throughout a game. This requires an emphasis on interval training and circuit exercises. The following plan details the full 12-week build-up to the start of the playing season. It is not uncommon for this programme to overlap into part of the season, or to start very soon after the end of the previous season (ensuring, of course, that you have a good 4-week rest after each season). Your resistance training should be in addition to this work.

Week	Frequency per week	Duration per session	Intensity % of MHR	Mode	Notes
1	3	30 min	75%	running or rowing	keep a high consistent pace
2	4	30-40 min	75-80%	run, step, row or cycle	as above
3	4	30-40 min	75-80%	as above	concentrate on running and stepping
4	2	40 min	70%	running	continuous effort
	2	30 min	90%	step, row or cycle	soft surfaces; intervals: 2 min at 90%, 2 min at 60% over 30 min

continued overleaf

Week	Frequency per week	Duration per session	Intensity % of MHR	Mode	Notes
5	as above	as above	as above	step or run	intervals and continuous all as above
6	1-2	20 min	40%	run, step or swim	rest week, keep light/stretching
7	1	30 min	60%	cycle, swim or row	continuous consistent pace
	1	40 min	85%	circuit	
	2	30-40 min	90%	interval sprints or running	1 min at 90%, 30 sec at 50%; work for 15 min, rest for 5 min and repeat for 15 min
8	as above	as above	as above	as above	as above
9	as above	as above	as above	as above	as above
10	as above	as above	as above	as above	as above
11	1	20-30 min	60%	swim, row, cycle or step	continuous activity
	1	40 min	85%	basketball circuit or aerobic classes	circuit
	1	20 min	90%	interval running	as week 7, work bout of 8 min only
12	as above	as above	as above	as above	as above

Basketball circuit

The circuit below can be used in conjunction with any circuit you are currently using. It should incorporate a comfortable mix of ballistic, jumping-type movements and lateral movements. Vary the time you work at each station, from 20 seconds to 1½ minutes. Transition time should be no more than 10 seconds between each exercise.

Station	Exercise	Notes
1	shuttle runs	run shuttles between 5-m marks
2	press-ups	combination of feet wide, close together, one foot raised, etc.
3	lateral shuttles	as for station 1, but use a defensive side shuffle for both left and right
4	knee tucks	use a mat, jumping and tucking the knees to the chest
5	crunch sit-ups	legs bent, back flat
6	burpees	squat, with palms on ground; push legs out behind, pull them in again and stand (or jump) up
7	lunge jumps	in a lunge position, jump and change legs
8	run on the spot	high knees and foot
9	half squat	ensure a full half-squat position with hands held above the head

The training week

Your training week may look as follows, depending on where in the 12-week programme you are:

Mon	aerobic and weights
Tues	intervals or circuits or rest
Wed	as for Monday and/or plyometrics
Thurs	as for Tuesday
Fri	as for Wednesday
Sat	rest or aerobic
Sun	rest

VOLLEYBALL

Volleyball can be played all year round, although there are distinct playing periods:

- the league season usually runs between September and April
- the tournament season between March and September
- the beach volleyball competition between June and August (in the northern hemisphere).

As one of the most popular participation sports, it is played on beaches and in parks in most countries of the world. On a competitive level there are 2 types of game: (1) beach volleyball and (2) the more traditional court (indoor) game.

Beach volleyball

With 2 players per team, the beach game requires each player to play in both positions. As it is often a fun sport, the game generally lacks the technical finesse and perfection of the indoor version!

Indoor court volleyball

The indoor game requires 6 players per team to be on court. These players rotate through the various court positions. One player is designated as the 'setter' and the remainder receive and hit the ball. All players must have the ability to 'block', which involves dynamic jumping, and be able to move explosively around the court with great agility and balance. As a team needs 2 clear points to win, the length of the game varies: most games last for at least 40 minutes, but can last as long as $1\frac{1}{2}$ hours. Points are won over short periods of very high-intensity work involving explosive lateral movements, jumping, hitting and short sprints over 2-5 m.

ENERGY SYSTEMS

Both beach and court games use primarily the short-burst anaerobic (ATP-CP) systems, as a point usually takes between 5-15 seconds to be played. Some top-level performers work for up to 30 seconds a point – that's hard work! The rest intervals are at the discretion of the serving team but are usually no longer than 20 seconds and can be as short as 5 seconds. The game is an explosive, power-based one which requires a good level of aerobic fitness to sustain such high-intensity anaerobic bursts. No one position has any physical requirements greater than or different to another. The only exception is the setter, who must have good shoulder and wrist flexibility and also an ability to sustain a 'hands above the head' position to facilitate 'setting' the ball for a large part of the game.

MUSCLES AND ACTIONS

Whether you are playing on the beach or on a court, you will be doing 2 fundamental things to hit and block the ball: jumping, and holding and moving your arms above your head. These skills, plus moving to the ball to return a serve or 'spike', place great emphasis on strength and explosive jumping ability. You use virtually every muscle in your legs, with a major responsibility falling on the buttocks, quadriceps and calf muscles. In receiving or hitting the ball, your arms are in constant use, with particular emphasis on the shoulder's rotator cuff muscles. The shoulder girdle muscles (deltoid, pectorals, latissimus dorsi, teres, and rhomboids in particular) and the abdominals are used constantly to stabilize the upper and lower body.

BENEFITS AND RISKS

Volleyball is particularly good for promoting muscle tone, especially in the legs. Your ability to sustain high-intensity interval work (anaerobic) is improved.

With such an explosive game, there are risks that may not be found in other team sports. Strains and sprains are not uncommon in the tendons, knee area and shoulder girdle. Such injuries occur to even the best-conditioned sportsperson. Finger injuries (ball strikes) are very common.

EQUIPMENT

For the indoor court game the essential pieces of equipment are shoes and knee and elbow pads. Buy specialized volleyball shoes that not only provide good lateral grip and support, but also help to reduce the chances of spraining an ankle. Because of the many diving, rolling and falling techniques used in returning the ball, knee and elbow pads are highly recommended. Shoes can be worn in the beach game but most participants prefer bare feet. Pads are not generally worn as the sand should be soft!

SPECIFIC STRETCHES

Both forms of volleyball require you to have good shoulder flexibility (and stability) as well as good hip, lower-leg and spinal rotation mobility. A good, general stretching routine should be complemented by the following specific exercises to be found in Chapter 6:

1. Standing calf.
2. Achilles tendon.
3. Chest and shoulder.
4. Front of hip.
5. Lower back.

ENTRY-LEVEL TRAINING

At this level the game is suited to all shapes and sizes. Social and fun beach games are sometimes mixed but more often segregated into 'guys' and 'girls' once a formal competition is undertaken. You need to have good basic fitness, good strength, a reasonable aerobic base and enough flexibility to use your skills. Volleyball is a skill-based sport and you will progress to advanced levels only if you increase your fitness along with your skills.

Good aerobic capacity and strength are essential to your explosive power. At entry level, consider playing one competition that will allow you to develop these aspects of your fitness in the first year. Doing this will ensure you do not play too much and injure yourself and will also allow you more time to focus on improving your game skills.

Activities: an overview

Weeks	Area of emphasis	Type of training
1-4	development of strength base and aerobic capacity	upper- and lower-body strength training; medium-distance continuous aerobic activities
5-8	muscle endurance in the lower body, strength in upper body; interval aerobic training	as above for weight training; aerobic-anaerobic circuit training with some continuous work
9	explosive leg power and continued upper-body power and endurance	elementary plyometric and jumping circuits
10-12	short initial aerobic training	anaerobic circuit training for game-specific conditioning
13	competition starts	

Work to a level that is comfortable for you and don't push yourself to the limit in every session. From week 5 onwards you will be in sufficient shape to work progressively harder, but for now work to around 80-90% of your maximum.

Aerobic conditioning: weeks 1-4

Week	Frequency per week	Duration (min)	Intensity	Details
1	2	15-20	70-75%	bike, swim, jog, row
2	3	20	60-75%	run, step or bike
3	3	30	70-80%	varied terrain running including small hills, step machine, row or swim
4	3	30	70-80%	as above

Resistance training: weeks 1-4

The following strength work is not too strenuous. You can do your resistance training on the same day as aerobic training (either before or after) or on alternate days:

Week	Sets	Reps	Rest between sets	Load % MHR	Frequency per week	Exercises
1	3	12	2 min	60% 1RM	1-2	all weeks: leg press, hamstring curl, bench press, lateral pull down, shoulder press, crunches
2	3	12	2 min	70% 1RM	1-2	
3	3	12-15	2 min	70% 1RM	2	
4	3	12-15	1 min	70-75%	2	

Aerobic training: weeks 5-8

Use the following aerobic circuit to accompany the recommended continuous training in this phase. Progress through A1, A2 and A3 as you get fitter. Begin by completing 2 circuits and progress up to working for 30 minutes (complete as many circuits as possible in this time).

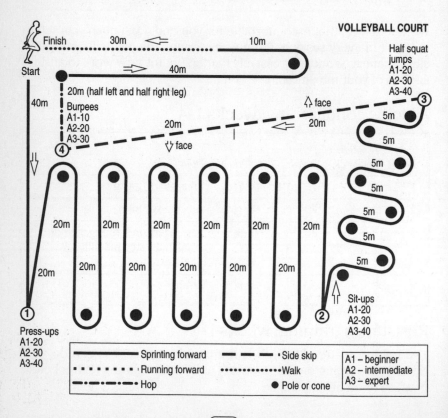

Week	Frequency per week	Duration (min)	Intensity	Details
5	2	30-40	70%	1 × circuit and 1 × either step or run
6	3	30-40	80%	1 × circuit and 2 × either run, row or step
7	3	30-40	85%	2 × circuit and 1 × run
8	3	30-40	85%	2 × circuit and 1 × run

Leg power: weeks 9-12

Over the previous 8 weeks you will have developed a good base level of aerobic capacity, strength and muscle endurance. Weeks 9-12 emphasize some of the more exacting movements and work-to-rest ratios seen in the game. Complete the weekly routine below:

Mon	complete the plyometric entry-level jump programme (page 76)
Tues	weights as weeks 5-8 but exclude leg exercises; upper body and abdominals only
Wed	continuous run, row, bike or swim for 30 min at 75% MHR
Thurs	as Mon
Fri	rest
Sat	as Tues plus a 30-min run or step
Sun	rest

After week 12, take a light week, training maybe once or twice before beginning to play the week after.

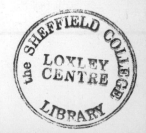
the SHEFFIELD COLLEGE
LOXLEY CENTRE
LIBRARY

·TRANSITION GOALS

Before you move into the advanced volleyball training section, you should be able to fulfil the following criteria. You should:

1. Not be suffering from any significant muscle or joint problems. If so, seek medical advice.
2. Be able to complete comfortably 30-plus minutes of continuous aerobic activity at 75% effort.
3. Have completed 6 weeks of regular resistance training.
4. Be able to complete 4-6 aerobic circuits (as above) comfortably.
5. Own good volleyball-specific shoes and pads in good repair.
6. Be reasonably proficient in the fundamental techniques of the game.
7. Eat regularly, with a diet including a minimum of 60% carbohydrate.
8. Drink a minimum of 4 pints of water a day.

ADVANCED-LEVEL TRAINING

Seriously competitive players are very explosive, very powerful and extremely agile. These qualities, combined with height, make top volleyball players (both men and women) among the most athletically conditioned of athletes. At advanced level you will:

- have to develop an excellent jumping ability, often over and above 80-90 cm
- have a low body fat, around 8-10% for men and 16-18% for women
- possess a competent array of playing skills
- be playing at least once a week and, quite possibly, twice a week on occasions

Before you can successfully maintain a year-round playing programme you will probably have to complete at least 1 or 2 seasons of serious conditioning training during an off-season period (between May and August). Only by doing this can you develop the necessary strength and power to see continued athletic progress and fully realize your potential.

Advanced aerobic conditioning: weeks 1-6

Week	Frequency per week	Duration (min)	Intensity % of max	Mode/terrain
1	3	30	75%	continuous row, run or step
2	3	40	80%	as week 1
3	4	40	60-85%	
4	4	50	60-85%	2 sessions as for week 1 and 2 sessions as for week 3
5	3	50	60-85%	as week 4
6	3	30	85%	20 min continuous running followed by 10 min of hill sprints: over 40 m at up to a 10% incline, jog back to start as recovery and repeat

Advanced resistance training: weeks 1-6

Week	Sets	Repetitions	Rest between sets (min)	Load %1RM	Frequency per week	Exercises
1	3-5	5-9	1	85%	3	single-leg press, single-leg curl, bench, lateral pull down, rotator cuff (see Chapter 9), shoulder press, crunches
2	3-5	5-9	1	85%	3	as week 1
3	3-5	5-9	2	85%	3	power cleans, bench press, dumbbell flys, lateral pull down, seated row, rotator cuff, crunches
4	3-5	5-9	2	85%	3	as week 3
5	3-5	5-9	3	90%	3	power cleans, dead lift (knees bent), dumbbell flys, lateral pull down, bench press, shoulder press, rotator cuff, crunches
6	3-5	5-9	3	90%	3	as week 5

Advanced aerobic conditioning: weeks 7-12

In this phase we concentrate primarily on explosive leg power through the use of plyometrics and related training methods (see Chapter 7). However, plyometrics will improve your explosive jump only in proportion to the basic strength you possess. You should ensure, therefore, that (1) you have a good strength base (especially in the legs) before you begin plyometric training and (2) that you continue (in the off-season) to build leg strength so that plyometric training will safely improve your jump and explosive power.

Week	Frequency per week	Duration (min)	Intensity	Mode/Terrain
7	3	30	60%	any choice of activity, e.g. swim, cycle, row but not running or high impact
8	3	30	85%	1 × week run or row, 2 × week 10-min jog and then run stairs or hills over 60-100 m; jog-back recovery and repeat for 15-20 min
9	3	30	85%	as week 8
10	3	30	85%	as week 8
11	3	30	85%	as week 8
12	1-2	20	60%	as week 7

As training is high impact (lots of jumping and working at near-maximum limits) there is a greater chance of minor injury. You must have a high intake of carbohydrate and fluids along with adequate rest if you are to complete the demands of training at this level.

Advanced power and resistance training: weeks 7-12

Week	Sets	Repetitions	Rest between sets (min)	Frequency per week	Exercises
7	see Chapter 7 for legs. Upper body 3 sets	30	2	2-3	2 × week plyometrics, 3 × week upper-body endurance; exercises as for weeks 1-6
8	as above				
9	as above				
10	as above				
11	as above				
12	rest week				no power or strength training

In conjunction with your resistance training over weeks 7-11, complete the plyometric advanced-level jump programme in Chapter 7. Remember always to stretch before and after this training and slowly progress from level to level over the 5-week period.

Training week for advanced-level conditioning (pre-season)

A typical week's training could look something like the following (specific volleyball training will be on top of this):

Mon	aerobic training
Tues	upper-body muscle endurance and plyometrics
Wed	aerobic training
Thurs	rest day
Fri	as for Tues
Sat	aerobic training
Sun	rest

CHAPTER 9

Racquet Sports

First, the obvious: all racquet sports are played with some type of racquet! Otherwise, racquet sports differ in the:

- type of court
- surface played on
- rules
- structure of game.

For example, tennis (the most popular racquet sport) and badminton are played indoors or outdoors on a divided court, over a net. Squash and racquetball are played on a shared court, against a wall and always indoors.

In physical terms, racquet sports are similar in that they:

- involve a stop-start, or intermittent, type of exercise
- have quite intense rallies separated by short recovery intervals
- involve running to a greater or lesser extent with the added involvement of the upper body. This is usually one-sided, although a two-handed shot is sometimes used.

SKILLS OVERVIEW

If you play one racquet sport regularly you are probably fairly proficient in another (tennis players often play squash in the winter and vice versa). The key skill here is good hand–eye co-ordination. On top of this you need a basic level of fitness and good tactical abilities. Hand–eye co-ordination is inherited (to a certain extent) but is also a skill that we learn as children. But don't be discouraged if you fall short in this area as it can always be improved with practice and patience. Also, a few lessons from a good instructor are invaluable and could help you discover hidden talent.

TRAINING OVERVIEW

Because of the similarities in the intermittent nature of all of these sports, there is much in common training-wise. Later in this chapter we provide a general-fitness programme for playing at entry level, followed by more specific, advanced programmes for reaching higher levels of proficiency. But first, let's examine what the demands and benefits are from each sport, and what are the important physical attributes you need to become a top professional or club player.

EQUIPMENT

Shoes

Due to the considerable amount of running around involved, wearing the correct shoes is very important. Shoes should have a good amount of cushioning to absorb continuous shocks. You may prefer to buy a good pair of trainers or running shoes that can be used for many sports and for the varied training sessions you will be doing. But make sure that they fit you well and are suitable for your specific type of training. Alternatively you may prefer to keep 1 pair of general trainers and a separate pair of tennis/squash/indoor trainers or court shoes.

The racquet

There is no right or wrong racquet: the choice is really down to your own personal preference.

- With tennis you can go for a jumbo-size, mid-size or standard-size head. The larger head makes it easier to hit the ball with the racquet's 'sweet spot'. Grip sizes vary.
- Badminton and racquetball are fairly standard so the choice is yours, depending on your budget. Grip sizes vary.
- With squash racquets, head sizes again vary so you must decide what size you feel most comfortable with. Grip sizes vary.

TENNIS

Tennis can be played strenuously or gently, depending on your skill level and that of your opponent. Those of you who want to can play all year round – there is a great range of floodlit, synthetic and indoor courts. These are particularly useful in winter when grass courts are unplayable. The game itself can last from 50 minutes to 2½ hours in women's singles, and from 2 to 5 hours in men's singles.

SOME GENERAL POINTS

Tennis rallies tend to be about the same duration as in squash. What makes tennis somewhat less strenuous, except at the top level, is the longer recovery between rally periods. Also, there are numerous breaks from play in tennis: between games, changing ends, preparing to hit or receive a serve, or retrieving the ball when it is out of play. Tennis rallies last, on average, from 4 to 10 seconds, depending on the type of court and the skill and fitness levels of the players. The work-to-rest ratio in tennis is 1:1.7. In other words, for every 1 second of play there are over 1½ seconds of recovery, which doesn't sound much but is actually quite generous.

HOW STRENUOUS IS TENNIS?

Tennis is an endurance sport in that, aerobically, it is approximately 88% demanding with only a 12% input required from anaerobic energy sources. The longer recovery periods reduce the overall intensity of the game, and you can expect to be working at about 50-60% of your maximum aerobic capacity in an average game. During a game you will be burning up a moderate 7-11 kilocalories per minute. A fairly tough hour-long match would probably use up close to 500 kilocalories (this figure would be lower in a game of doubles).

Heart rate

Despite the stop-and-start nature of tennis, your heart rate during a match will remain at about 70% of your maximum heart rate (except when changing ends). For the average person this would be about 150 beats per minute.

Fitness levels

The moderate intensity of the game at recreational level allows you to play tennis if your fitness level is low. If you are reasonably fit, however, tennis is not very effective in further improving your aerobic fitness. Naturally, if you are very competitive and play regularly against strong opposition, your tennis game could be far more strenuous. Bear in mind that a good level of fitness is advantageous towards the end of a match when, inevitably, reaction times slow up and you anticipate less effectively and lose concentration.

The muscles used

It is during the fast rallies that the majority of the work is done in tennis and this is where quick reaction times, speedy and flexible footwork, and fast arm movements become important. The running nature of the game involves all the major muscles in your legs, while serving and hitting the ball involve your shoulder muscles and those in the back and front of the upper racquet arm (the triceps and biceps).

PLAYER PROFILE

Success in recreational and club tennis is very dependent on skill. At top levels, however, there tends to be a narrowing in skill levels. Some players give themselves an edge through fast reaction times or a powerful serve. Others may be fitter, although this fitness advantage may show only at the end of a match when fewer unforced errors are made. Also, a positive mental attitude helps players at all levels deal with match pressure and regain confidence after a break of serve or a few lost points.

Height

Generally, good tennis players tend to be reasonably tall. Male international players are 178-183 cm and female international players are 163-168 cm. Height is an advantage for developing a strong serve and, of course, when reaching for volleys and lobs. If you are a tall person you also tend to be more intimidating at the net! However, to be a really valuable asset, height must be accompanied by strength and power. Tennis players tend to be relatively muscular but lean with it.

Body fat

At the top level of play, body-fat levels are about 11-15% (men) and 18-20% (women). There is a very distinct difference in body-fat levels in county- and club-level female tennis players. Female county players have an average of 19% body fat and female club players a staggering 28%, which is about the average for healthy inactive people. Slightly lowering body fat, therefore, will help you achieve a better standard of tennis.

Aerobic fitness

Top male players have VO_2 max levels of 50-60 ml/kg/min while females have levels of 43-48 ml/kg/min. A high aerobic capacity is not necessarily a prerequisite for success in tennis, although it does help the higher up the ladder you go.

SQUASH

Squash is another hugely popular racquet sport. It is, in fact, the third most regularly played sport in Britain (behind swimming and badminton, and not counting walking). As an indoor sport, squash is played all year round, although the 'season' is officially between May and September. International squash players have a busy itinerary as they also tend to be on county or provincial teams and move from tournament to tournament with club matches slotted in between. The duration of the game is usually 30-60 minutes at recreational and club level while international players can play 5-game matches lasting up to 3 hours.

Remember that squash, at all levels, is not a 'gentle' game. This is especially true for those of you with a competitive streak! This has important ramifications if you are unfit, overweight or have any medical problems. You definitely must be fit before you start to play squash.

HOW DEMANDING IS SQUASH?

The work-to-rest ratio in squash is about 1:1 (tennis has almost double the rest period). The average length of time for a rally is about 7 seconds, with a small percentage lasting longer than 20 seconds. While on the court, you can expect to be active for about half the duration of the match. The other half is spent collecting the ball and returning to the serve-or-receive position. You are therefore playing for 15 minutes of a 30-minute game, whereas in tennis you may play for only 5 minutes of a 30-minute game.

Aerobic demands

Squash is a very strenuous game as your heart rate is usually at about 80-90% of your maximum, which is very high. It places large demands on your stamina and lung capacity. In energy terms, club and recreational players probably burn up about 700 kilocalories in an hour-long game exercising at 60-75% of maximum aerobic capacity. Although squash involves repeated fast bursts and could be judged an anaerobic-type sport, the short recovery time between rallies definitely makes huge demands on the aerobic system. Having good aerobic fitness helps you recover between points and maintain your speed around the court.

The muscles used

In squash your legs have to work very hard getting you around the court. This involves the quadriceps, the hamstrings and the calf muscles. There is no great arm swing as in tennis or badminton; the squash stroke is more a flick of the wrist. But a strong upper body, and forearm in particular, will put more power behind your shots.

Fluid loss

You should be aware that you can lose a lot of fluid during a game. Have you noticed how much some players sweat during a tough game? You may sweat up to 2 litres of fluid in an hour – no small amount. When you lose this amount your body can start to overheat, so it is extremely important to drink plenty of water after a game and, if possible, drink small amounts of water during the game.

PLAYER PROFILE

Height

Unlike tennis, squash is not a sport in which height is an advantage: competitive players tend to be of average height.

Body fat

As fast movements around the court are important, excess body fat will be a disadvantage. Male squash players tend to have 10-12% body fat as compared to 16-18% on the average person of the same age. From club to county standard there is a dramatic difference in body-fat levels, particularly in women. Regular club players tend to have a body-fat level of about 25% compared to levels below 16% often found in county players. This is almost certainly due to the increase in training as competition gets tougher.

Aerobic fitness

Due to the highly demanding nature of the game, squash players have to be very fit. The average VO_2 max level for males is 60-64 ml/kg/min and for females 52-56 ml/kg/min. Again, fitness improves from recreational, to club and up to county level. A recreational player may expect to have a VO_2 max of about 42-46 ml/kg/min. To step up to county standard the VO_2 max would have to increase to 50-54 ml/kg/min.

BADMINTON

Badminton, often considered a 'gentle' game, can be played by people of all levels of fitness. Competitive badminton, however, can be a highly explosive and skilled sport. Although the badminton court is smaller than a tennis court, the net is higher (1.55 m), requiring a good proportion of overhead shots.

HOW STRENUOUS IS BADMINTON?

A match lasts about 36-45 minutes and consists of 3 sets. When playing, say, a 36-minute match you will be actively playing for a third of this time (more than tennis and less than squash). The size of the court and the time spent retrieving the shuttlecock and returning to the serving position account for some of this difference. The average length of a rally in badminton is very similar at all levels of play, at about 4-5 seconds. The recovery period can be anywhere from 5-10 seconds, again falling in between those for squash and tennis.

Fitness levels

An interesting fact is that the amount of energy used during a game of badminton is lower than in tennis, even though badminton appears more demanding. This could be because it is played on a smaller court and there is less ground to cover and because tennis uses more upper-body muscles. Kilocalories burnt up in badminton increase from 6 per minute for recreational players to 10 per minute at club level. This is even higher at international levels. A moderate 40-minute match, therefore, would burn up around 240 kilocalories (lower in doubles).

Heart rate

Heart rates are generally higher in badminton than in tennis. If you play regularly, you can expect yours to be around 70% of your maximum heart rate. If you are highly skilled it could increase to 80% of your max.

Muscles used

Badminton involves a lot of leg-muscle action, especially with the calf muscles. The overhead arm action is more of a wrist than a shoulder movement and any power would be more likely to come from the strong shoulders and forearms, rather than the arms.

Flexibility

The high proportion of overhead work in badminton requires you to be extremely flexible. To reduce the risk of a strained muscle as you reach for the shuttlecock, you should include a thorough stretching routine as part of your preparation.

PLAYER PROFILE

Height and body fat

There is not an ideal height or weight in badminton. Body-fat levels tend to be close to the average, moderately active individual. But, as you might expect, body-fat levels decrease as the standard of play increases from club up to county and international levels.

Aerobic fitness

Generally, badminton players tend to be fitter than tennis players. The average VO_2 max value in international players is about 59-64 ml/kg/min (men) and 50-54 ml/kg/min (women). Naturally these are the highest levels – you can certainly play a good game of badminton with lower levels. But a superior aerobic capacity in a game like badminton will ensure that your opponent tires quicker than you do.

RACQUETBALL

Racquetball is similar to squash but although it can be played on a squash court it is usually played on a slightly larger court. The ball is about the size of a tennis ball and is more 'bouncy' than a squash ball (hence the use of the ceiling in racquetball). The racquet has a relatively large head and is short-handed.

HOW STRENUOUS IS RACQUETBALL?

As in squash, about half the game time is spent in actual play, with rallies lasting an average of 10-15 seconds. The work-to-rest ratio is about 1:2, making racquetball slightly easier than squash. But bear in mind that there is more ground to cover and the lively ball makes it quite a fast game.

Heart rate

The intensity or pace of the game is similar to that of squash, with an average heart rate of 70-80% of the maximum. Interestingly, in any of these tactical racquet sports there can be an enormous difference in the heart rates of 2 opponents. This is because the better or more skilful player can have the other running all over the court. It is not unusual in racquetball to have one player with a reasonably strenuous heart rate of 145 bpm while the other player tears frantically around the court with his or her heart pumping at 180 beats per minute.

Fitness levels

The average amount of energy burnt in racquetball is 10-14 kilocalories per minute. This increases as the standard improves from beginner to advanced.

PLAYER PROFILE

Height and body fat

Players of both racquetball and squash are generally similar in height and weight. Top-level racquetball players tend to be quite lean with body-fat levels of about 8-12% (men) and 14% (women). This is lower than those for tennis and badminton since racquetball is a more strenuous game and requires a greater amount of fitness training.

Aerobic capacity

Aerobic capacity is similar to that of squash players, with VO_2 max levels of 50-56 ml/kg/min (men) and 40-46 ml/kg/min (women).

TRAINING FOR RACQUET SPORTS

Flexibility

All racquet sports require good flexibility:

- For quick side-to-side, lateral mobility you need good adductor (inner-thigh) flexibility.
- Explosive forward and backward movements require you to have good ranges of movement in the hamstrings, thighs and, most significantly, the calf.
- Excellent mobility in the shoulder and the ability to twist (spinal rotation) at your mid-section are also essential.

In addition to the general-flexibility exercises in your warm-up, you should also perform the exercises suggested below.

Stretches for flexibility

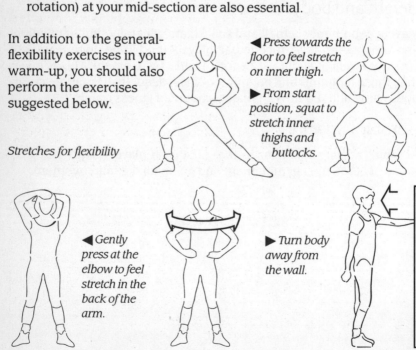

◄ *Press towards the floor to feel stretch on inner thigh.*

► *From start position, squat to stretch inner thighs and buttocks.*

◄ *Gently press at the elbow to feel stretch in the back of the arm.*

► *Turn body away from the wall.*

Physical demands of racquet sports

Sport	Work-to-rest ratio	Length of average rally	Time in actual play per 30 min	Top aerobic levels male	Top aerobic levels female	Calories burnt per min
tennis	1:1.7	4-10 sec	5-10	50-60	43-48	7-10
squash	1:1.0	4-14 sec	13-15	60-64	52-56	10-12
badminton	1:1.4	4-6 sec	8-10	59-64	50-54	10-11
raquetball	1:2.0	10-15 sec	15-17	50-56	40-46	10-14

Aerobic training

Aerobic demand is similar across racquet sports. The levels quoted in the above table are for the top-level players: recreational-player levels would be some 10-12 points lower. To enable you to get the most out of playing, you should look to a 5-week build-up before you begin. This is important especially for particularly demanding games such as racquetball and squash in which it is difficult to play an 'easy' game. This brings us back to the 'be fit to play' philosophy rather than the 'play to get fit' approach.

Your aerobic work should cover a range of activities. All of the racquet games require good running ability, so some of your activity should be running oriented, preferably on a variety of terrains. Add in some slight hills – undulating, soft-impact ground such as a golf course is particularly suitable. Stepping, cross-country, ski machines and the like are also very useful. Follow the time and intensity guidelines below over your first 5 weeks:

Aerobic training: weeks 1-5

Week	Intensity (% of MHR)	Duration (min)	Notes
1	60%	20	all of these times can be covered at a jog if you are new to any of the games
2	60-65%	20-25	
3	75-80%	25-30	
4	75-80%	30-35	
5	75-80%	40-45	

Entry-level court drills

Once you begin playing you will discover muscles you had no idea existed and you will not be able to avoid post-exercise soreness. This often occurs when you perform an unfamiliar exercise at a higher level than you are used to. To counteract this, and to make your training even more specific, it is a good idea to include some court drills in your routine. There are many of these drills and most have a skill component to them.

When using court drills, begin gently. Start by completing a set of 4 repetitions and rest for approximately 2-3 times as long as it takes you to complete one repetition. For example, if it takes you 20 seconds to do 1 repetition, you should rest for 40-60 seconds before you go on to the next drill. After a set of 4, rest, and stretch for 4-5 minutes. You should complete 3-4 sets of 4 repetitions in each drill. This means your training time will be about 35-40 minutes.

Tennis drill

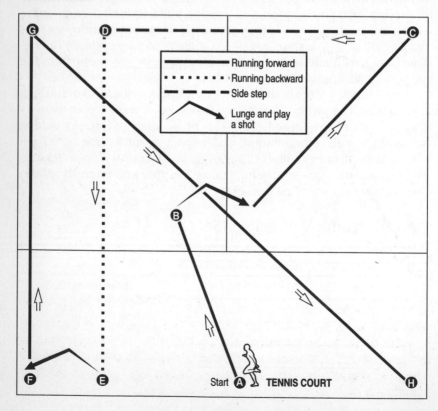

Running forward
Running backward
Side step
Lunge and play a shot

Start Ⓐ TENNIS COURT

Start at A, sprint forward to B, lunge to your right and play an imaginary shot (carrying your racquet, of course!). Now sprint to the net at point C. From here, shuffle across the net as if you had to make a volley at D. Now back peddle (run backwards) to E, and make a shot as if to get a lob. At E lunge to the left, as if to play a shot (F), then sprint forwards again to G, finally turning round to sprint to H. This type of drill is obviously longer than a rally: it is designed to be so. It also has the turning, twisting and sideways movements you use in the game.

Squash and racquetball drill

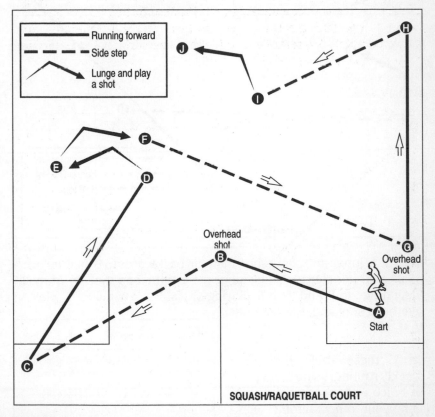

Start at A, sprint to B and play an overhead shot. Side shuffle to C, sprint to D and lunge to the left, playing a shot (E). Immediately lunge to the right and play a shot (F), then side step to G and play another overhead shot. Sprint to H, side step back and then lunge to the left, playing a shot.

Badminton drill

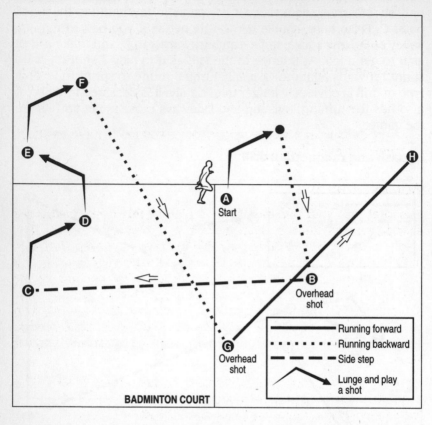

BADMINTON COURT

Start at A, lunge and play a shot, then run backwards to B. Play an overhead shot, side step to C, then lunge to the right for a shot (D). Immediately lunge to E and then F, playing shots. Back pedal to G, play an overhead shot and, finally, sprint to H.

Work these drills into your weekly routine, using them once or twice a week in conjunction with your other aerobic work. Your week could look as follows:

Mon	aerobic
Tues	drills and short game
Wed	aerobic
Thurs	drills
Fri	rest
Sat	play
Sun	optional

ADVANCED-LEVEL TRAINING

At this level we assume you are serious about your game. At this point in your preparation you should note the following:

1. Resistance training is an important factor, especially for leg development. Good upper-body strength is an advantage but superior leg strength is vital if you are to develop an explosive ability on the court.
2. Court drills must become very intense. You really have to attack them with everything you've got!

Aerobic training

It is vital that your aerobic ability is high at this level. Rallies are shorter but very intense, often pushing you to your maximum. The only way to recover quickly from such high-intensity bouts of effort is to have a high VO_2 max to clear the waste products (lactic acid, etc.) built up during a rally. Get on your bike, the step machine or the rower, or swim or run. You need lots of variety but all exercise must be continuous and steady. The variety helps cut down the load on your legs as they will be severely tested during your game-specific fitness work. You must be able to cope with 3 aerobic sessions per week:

1st session: At 60-65% of your MHR and to last for at least 50-60 minutes but preferably up to 90 minutes.
2nd session: 40 minutes at over 75% of your MHR.
3rd session: 25-30 minutes at over 85% of your MHR.

Resistance training

Leg strength is vital if you wish to be more explosive and is fundamental to plyometric work. If new to resistance training you should follow the entry-level programme for strength training (7-9 repetitions) in Chapter 5. Those of you who have concentrated primarily on your aerobic fitness without much emphasis on strength should also follow the entry-level programme. Those familiar with weight training can begin with the advanced exercises. Remember that it is important to retain your agility, so bulk is not what you require. Persist with strength routines and avoid those that emphasize muscle bulk. Bear in mind, however, that some bulk (or redefinition) will always occur when you weight train.

Although not exclusive to racquet sports, there is a correlation between playing racquet sports and shoulder instability. This occurs as one set of muscles, usually those in your front shoulder and chest, become stronger than those in the back. This can result in a weak 'rotator cuff'. The rotator-cuff group of muscles stabilize and control the fine movement in your shoulder. The stronger chest and shoulder muscles (developed through playing and training) can overpower these 'deeper' muscles in the shoulder. We strongly suggest you do some rotator-cuff exercises as a preventative measure against shoulder instability. This is imperative if you have already experienced problems.

In each of these exercises, do 8-10 repetitions per set and complete 1-3 sets. If using a rubber exercise band, remember to attach one end to something solid, ensuring the connection is secure.

Rotator-cuff exercises

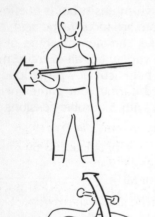

Keeping your upper arm close to the side and your elbow at a right angle, hold on to a rubber exercise band (or cable weight machine).

Pull the band by turning your forearm outwards.

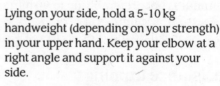

Lying on your side, hold a 5-10 kg handweight (depending on your strength) in your upper hand. Keep your elbow at a right angle and support it against your side.

Lift weight towards the ceiling and slowly lower back down.

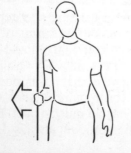

Stand with your upper arm close to your side, elbow at a right angle and the back of your hand against a wall.

Push the back of your hand against the wall. Hold for approximately 10 seconds.

continued

164

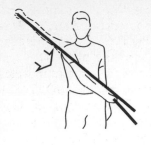

Stand with your arm down and out to the side. Hold on to a rubber exercise band (or cable weight machine).

Pull the band up and across your body, letting your thumb lead the movement.

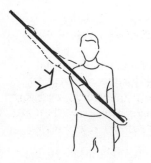

Stand or sit with the hand of the arm to be exercised on your opposite hip. Hold on to a rubber exercise band (or cable weight machine).

Pull the band up towards the opposite side.

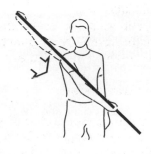

Stand with your arm up and out to the side. Hold on to a rubber exercise band (or cable weight machine).

Pull the band down and across your body, letting your thumb lead the movement.

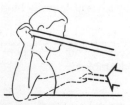

Sit on a chair with your arm lifted out to the side and elbow at a right angle supported on a table. Hold on to a rubber exercise band which is in front of you.

Pull the band, keeping your elbow bent and resting on the table.

continued

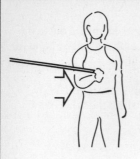

Keeping your upper arm close to the side and elbow at a right angle, hold on to a rubber exercise band (or cable weight machine).

Pull the band towards your stomach.

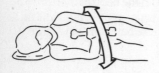

Lying on your side, hold a 5-10 kg handweight in the hand lying on the floor. Keep the elbow at a right angle and support it against your side.

Lift weight towards the ceiling and lower back down.

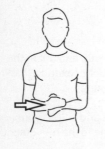

Stand with your arm close to your side and your elbow at a right angle.

Push the palm of your hand against the other hand. Hold for approximately 10 seconds.

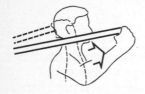

Sit on a chair with your arm lifted to the side and your elbow at a right angle supported on a table. Hold on to a rubber exercise band which is fastened behind you.

Pull the band, keeping your elbow bent and resting on the table.

Pre-season preparation training: weekly routine, weeks 6-8

Mon	strength training and rotator cuff
Tues	aerobic: 50-60 min
Wed	as for Monday
Thurs	aerobic: 25-30 min
Fri	as for Monday
Sat	aerobic: 40 min
Sun	rest

The late pre-season

With 4-6 weeks to the start of your competitive period you should reduce the amount of longer-distance aerobic work and cut out all lower-body (leg) resistance training. Continue your rotator-cuff exercises year round and emphasize leg power and game-specific drills. Your weekly training routine could look as follows. Remember that your skill training will need to be accommodated around this work.

Mon	aerobic session: rotate between 50-60 min for 1 session, 25-30 min for the next, 40 min for the next, and so on.
Tues	plyometrics and court drills
Wed	upper-body strength and light aerobic: 30 min 70% MHR
Thurs	plyometrics and court drills
Fri	rest
Sat	optional
Sun	upper-body strength

Plyometric training

This work will really improve your off-the-spot acceleration. You should emphasize every explosive movement over 2-5 m. Cover distances of only 5 m in the 'running' drills. If you are unfamiliar with some of the drills or new to plyometrics, you must use the entry-level acceleration programme. Over several weeks you should be able to move on to some of the advanced acceleration programme exercises. See Chapter 7 on plyometrics for training details.

Advanced-level court drills

Tennis

1. Complete 6-8 repetitions per set of the entry-level drill. Rest for exactly 1.7 times the time it takes you to complete a repetition (that is, 10 seconds' work equals 17 seconds' rest before the next repetition). Complete 3 sets and rest for 3½ minutes between sets.
2. Move on to the drill below. Complete the same number of repetitions per set (6-8), the same number of sets (3) and work to the same work-to-rest ratio of 1:1.7.

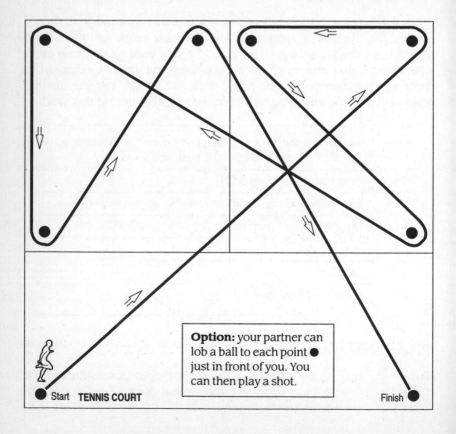

Option: your partner can lob a ball to each point ● just in front of you. You can then play a shot.

Start **TENNIS COURT**

Finish

Squash and racquetball

Squash: Do the advanced and entry-level drills. Complete 4 repetitions per set. Complete 4-6 sets. Rest for exactly the same time as it takes you to complete each repetition, e.g. 15 seconds' work to 15 seconds' rest. Practise 1-3 minutes' rest (stretching) between sets. This is a tough workout if you give it 100%.

Racquetball: Use the same drills with a work-to-rest ratio of 1:2. The difference in court size should ensure your work interval is slightly longer. If you play on a squash court then you're lucky! Your rest interval is twice as long as the work period, e.g. 15 seconds' work to 30 seconds' rest.

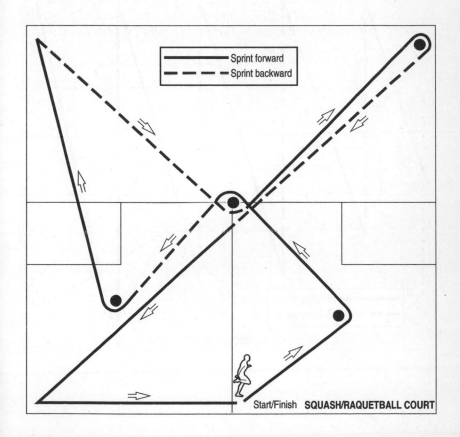

Badminton

Although the play periods are quite short in badminton, they are often close together. To ensure you get a good training effect it is very important that you concentrate on moving quickly from one repetition to the next, as you could easily overrun your rest interval. Use the advanced and entry-level drills. Complete 12 repetitions of each drill per set. Complete 2-3 sets of each. Walk to the start between repetitions, using this as your rest. Rest for 1-3 minutes between sets.

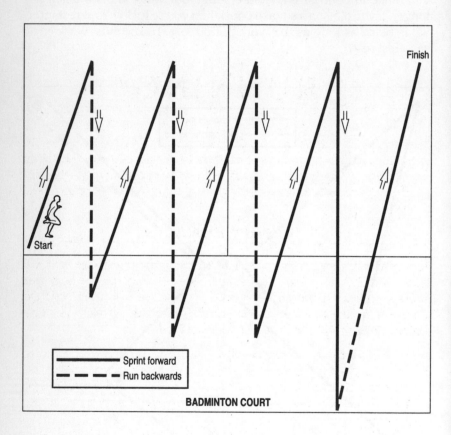

BADMINTON COURT

CHAPTER 10

Individual Sports

RUNNING

This section looks at the most popular running distances for beginners: from road races of 3 km to marathons. It tells you how your body works when you're running and takes you from preparing for your first road race to more structured and rigorous preparation for a marathon.

WHY RUN?

Road racing is one of the most versatile of sports, and one that just about anyone can enjoy. There are events throughout the year and there's always a great variety of races to choose from, although the choice is naturally wider in the summer months. As well as being enjoyable, running can bring the following benefits:

- Joints, muscles and ligaments become more flexible.
- Your heart, itself a muscle, begins to work more efficiently with your lungs. More blood is sent to your lungs or muscles with every heartbeat. Both your exercise and resting heart rate may decrease by 20% or even more.
- A more efficient heart leads to more blood flow to the kidneys, so they function better, too.
- The shape of your legs can improve, with less fat and better muscle definition.
- You become trimmer all round as muscles firm up.
- Your ability to regulate your body temperature improves. You sweat more to cool down efficiently and find you can tolerate heat better.

Because of all these potential benefits, running is a great way to improve your general fitness for many sports: running sessions feature in many of the sport-specific programmes in this book. If you are a regular and reasonably fit runner, you'll be basically fit enough to have a go at most sports, if you fancy a change.

> Running can help you stop smoking. If you don't give up immediately, you will probably feel the need to cut down, and eventually you are likely to give up completely. Of new runners, only 7% still smoke after 6 months.

HOW YOU RUN

Here's some information about how your body works when you run. It's worth understanding some of this so you can appreciate what is happening and what problems may arise.

Muscles for running

When you run, your quadriceps (the muscles on the front of your thigh) and shins are the workhorses, while your hamstrings (muscles at the back of the legs) help you slow down or stop. The quadriceps and hamstrings are both vital to the movement of your knees. Because of the enormous power output of hamstrings during sprinting, they are easily torn or pulled, particularly if not properly warmed up.

Moving your hip involves at least two muscles, the gluteus maximus at the back (buttocks) and the iliopsoas at the front.

The two large muscles that form the calf muscle, the gastrocnemius and the soleus, help you to flex your ankle during running.

Your upper body does less work in running, but relaxed shoulders and a smooth arm movement help create a smooth running action, as well as propelling you forward when going uphill or running fast.

ENERGY TO RUN

During the first few minutes of running you are producing energy anaerobically. This can give you an uncomfortable feeling in your legs and make you feel slightly breathless. A beginner often gives up at this stage but, if you keep going just a little longer and allow your body to settle into its normal rhythm the exercise will begin to feel more comfortable.

Once you reach a comfortable, steady pace, you start to burn more fat than carbohydrate and produce energy aerobically. The fitter you are, the higher the proportion of fat you will use during steady running. This is an advantage as your body's stores of fat are far greater than those of carbohydrate.

Burning calories and 'the wall'

Very roughly, you burn about 100 kilocalories per mile while running; it varies with your body weight. You can calculate how much energy you burn for your own body weight using the table in Appendix 2.

However, you can store enough glycogen (carbohydrate stored in the muscles or liver) for only about 90 minutes of exercise – even on a well-balanced, high-carbohydrate diet. After this, you must slow down as your body starts to burn more fat, which releases energy more slowly than carbohydrate. This partly explains the feeling of reaching 'the wall' which marathon runners often talk about. The wall is commonly explained as the point at which your carbohydrate stores run so low that your body has to switch over to fat as the main fuel source. You can delay this by drinking a carbohydrate-containing sports drink (during a long run). Some runners describe the feeling as being similar to treading water or having heavy legs. In endurance races such as marathons almost all runners have to slow down. The winner is usually the one who slows down the least.

WHAT TO AIM FOR

The distance of most races these days is given in kilometres, but the training distances are usually given in miles as this is still in common usage. For convenience, think of 10 km as 6 miles, or 1 km as 0.6 of a mile.

In any sport, it is always easier to train if you have a goal in mind – this could be to run 2, 5, or 10 miles without stopping – but to train with a real race in mind is even better. There are running races of all standards to choose from.

Fun run

Ideal for a newcomer is a fun run over 3-5 km, and there are plenty to choose from. Look through some sports or running magazines, or even the local paper, and pick a race that's about 3 months ahead. The entry-level training programme below will take you through training for a 5-km (3.1-mile) fun run.

10-km run

If you already run and feel you could aim higher than a fun run, the next distance to aim for is a 10-km run. There are tips on adjusting the training programme for a 10-km race after the entry-level section below.

Marathon

The marathon is an endurance event which has become enormously popular all over the world and provides an attainable challenge for many runners. A marathon is 26 miles 385 yards (42.2 km). Elite runners take just over 2 hours to complete this distance at speeds of 11-12 mph. You don't even need to run a marathon particularly well to achieve great personal satisfaction. Once you've done it, though, the desire to improve spurs you on to do another – and improve your time.

MARATHON RUNNER PROFILE

Here is the profile of a typical elite male marathon runner. Don't worry if you don't match up to it. You can still run marathons effectively and in good times:

Average height:	170 cm (although many are smaller).
Typical weight:	61 kg, with a low body-fat level of about 4-8%.
Age:	Best marathon performances recorded by people in their late 30s and early 40s.
Fitness:	They tend to have a high maximum aerobic capacity (over 75 ml/kg/min) and can run at a high percentage of this capacity. They often have a lot of a particular type of muscle fibre called 'slow twitch endurance fibre': 79%, compared to 58% in an untrained person. This is partly genetic and partly due to training.

WHAT TO WEAR

Running is ideal for beginners as you don't need a lot of expensive equipment.

Running shoes

A good pair of shoes is essential, but you needn't pay the earth for them. There are numerous brands of running shoes on the market and each has its own special feature, designed to make you go faster or the shoes last longer. You simply need to find a shoe that suits your feet and the amount of running you intend to do. Here are some considerations to help you choose:

1. The main difference between shoe brands is the shape. Try different makes to find out which one suits your foot shape best.
2. You will need very different shoes if you are running casually twice a week from those you will need if you are doing a regular 40 miles per week of road pounding. A good sports-shop assistant should be able to help you choose the right pair for your needs.
3. You need good shock absorption in the heel and mid-shoe flexibility to allow your foot to bend. Again, try the shoe to see how easily it bends and ask an assistant to advise you.
4. Don't spend a fortune or go for the top of the range. Stick to a sensible basic shoe with a known brand name. You can always upgrade.
5. Aim to replace shoes every 6 months or 600 miles, whichever comes first.

Clothes

What you wear is up to you, and the weather. It is best to wear loose clothing and, especially in winter, wear several light layers. This allows heat to evaporate and your skin to breathe more easily. You can remove layers as you warm up. Running tights or tracksters (light, close-fitting track bottoms) are better than heavy, baggy tracksuit bottoms. Women runners need to invest in a good-quality sports bra. Cotton-and-nylon-mix socks are better than plain cotton ones – cotton retains the sweat, which evaporates more quickly with nylon. Suitable clothes are available from most sports shops.

WHERE TO RUN

The best surface to run on is firm, relatively flat and smooth, with some shock absorption. For example, a pavement can be too hard, but a running track has a lot more 'give'. Grass is softer and less jarring on your joints but can make your muscles and tendons work harder; there's also a danger of injury as the ground can be uneven. The best option is to vary the surface you run on – alternate between road, grass, trails and treadmills.

ENTRY-LEVEL TRAINING: 5 KM OR 10 KM

Before you start the training programme below, here are a few things you need to know:

Stretching

Runners should ideally stretch before and after a run, but if time is limited the after-run stretch is the most important. Pre-run stretches should be gentle. After the run, when the muscles are warmer and looser, hold the stretch longer and extend the movement a little further.

The most important muscles to stretch are the calf muscles and the back and front of the thigh muscles as these are the main ones used in running. Try these stretching exercises from Chapter 6:

1. Quadriceps stretch
2. Hamstring stretch
3. Calf stretch
4. Achilles tendon stretch.

Pre-training

Whatever your reason for starting to run, your first target is to get your body used to running regularly, whatever the speed. Try to get up to jogging for 15 minutes continuously, at whatever speed is comfortable for you, by the end of two weeks. Don't worry if you can't do it. Complete your 15 minutes by walking and jogging, gradually trying to reduce the amount of walking. Once you can complete 15 minutes of continuous jogging, you are ready to start the entry-level training programme.

Training for 5 km

This programme will prepare you for a 5-km fun run. For each week of preparation, there may be a specific time and/or distance to run and frequency of runs during the week. If just a time is given, run at any speed, with no set distance in mind, speeding up or slowing down as suits you. Runs like this will become your long, slow distance runs (LSD) as you progress. The aim of these is to choose a comfortable pace and just enjoy yourself. Always warm up before the paced runs (week 6 onwards). The programme starts off gently but gets quite tough in weeks 7-12. At the end of the 12-week programme, you should be able to manage 4 miles and be able to run continuously for 45 minutes, which will make a 5-km fun run an easy target.

Week	Distance (miles)	Duration (min)	Frequency per week
1	any distance (LSD)	18	4
2	any distance (LSD)	20	2
	1	10	2
3	any distance (LSD)	22	2
	1½	15	2
4	2	20	2
	1	9½	2
5	any distance (LSD)	23	2
	1½	14	2
6	2	19	2
	2 × 1 mile (3-min rest between)	9+9	2
7	any distance (LSD)	25	2
	2	18	2
8	2 × 1 mile + 1 × ½ mile (1-min rest between)	9+9+5	2
	any distance (LSD)	25	3
9	3 × 1 mile (2-min rest between)	9+9+9	2
	any distance (LSD)	27	2

continued

Week	Distance (miles)	Duration (min)	Frequency per week
10	any distance (LSD)	30	2
	3	28	2
11	any distance (LSD)	35	2 or 3
	3½	any time	2
12	any distance (LSD)	40-45	2
	4	38	2

If you find the increase from one week to another too much at any stage, either stay on the same schedule for an extra week or cut the increase in the time or distance by half.

Getting hooked

Whether you run a race or not, the next step is to ask yourself:

1. Do you just want to maintain the same level of fitness, doing the occasional fun run or road race? If so, that's fine. Just follow the same format, repeating weeks 10-12, running 4 or 5 days per week. You could split your runs like this:
   - 1 or 2 longer runs (LSD)
   - 2 shorter runs, where you try to keep up a good pace and stretch yourself a bit (anything from 2 to 4 miles)

   Or
   - Try progressively increasing the time for 1 of your long runs by adding about 2 minutes each week.

2. Or are you hooked? Do you want to move on to longer distances? To keep improving, start to incorporate some interval, or paced, training, like this:
   - Add 5 to 10 bursts of 10-30 seconds of fast running in the middle of your run when you are well warmed up. Allow about 1 minute of easy jogging to recover between bursts.

Do your long run at the weekend, in a park or anywhere with varied terrain. Set a relaxed and 'sociable' pace – and see if you can persuade a friend to join you.

178

If you decide to keep up your running, it's worth finding out about a local road-running club. There are plenty around and they cater for all levels.

Training for 10 km

If you would like to stretch yourself a bit more, the next distance to aim for is a 10-km race. To train for this, follow the entry-level programme but make the following changes:

- Allow 6 weeks for training. Start at week 10 of the entry-level programme.
- After entry-level week 12 gradually increase the length of your runs by adding about 5 minutes or ½ mile each week.
- Add some intervals once you are well warmed up. For example, include several 2- to 6-minute faster-pace runs with 1-2 minutes' active recovery between (that means keep jogging). Do longer bursts on longer runs.

Training tips

- Slower running educates the muscles to work more efficiently, in an aerobic way.
- Pick up the pace towards the end of a run to get the optimum training effect.
- Try 1 long run per week, perhaps on Saturday or Sunday, or split this up into 2 shorter ones if you find it too difficult.
- Always cool down after a run by slowing down the pace gradually to an easy jog and then a walk.

TRANSITION GOALS

Before you consider moving on to the next section to train for a marathon, answer these questions:

1. Can you run 3 miles in 27 minutes?
2. Can you run continuously for 40 minutes?
3. Do you have suitable running shoes that are not more than 1 year old?
4. Are you free from injuries or unusual pains in your knees or back?
5. Are you aware of the need for carbohydrate in your diet and do you know which foods to get it from?

6. Do you drink plenty of non-alcoholic drinks (more than 3 pints of water per day)?

If you can answer yes to all of these questions you should be ready to tackle the big challenge of the marathon. If not, wait a few weeks until you are ready to move on. You may already have done a marathon but now want to focus your training more and improve your time. The advanced schedule below is geared towards completing a marathon in about 4½ hours.

ADVANCED-LEVEL TRAINING: MARATHON

This schedule should be started 6½ months before the marathon – you should reach week 24 about 2 weeks before the race. Work back from the date of the race to find when you should start training.

Allow 1-2 minutes' recovery between repetitions. Training is given for 2 weeks together. Some weeks have 2 longer runs of different durations. The training weeks are divided between time and distance targets. Running for pace/distance is not a main concern; distance/ pace is given as a recommended time to cover the given distance.

Weeks	Distance (miles)	Duration/pace (min)	Frequency per week
1 + 2	any distance	30 (week 1); 40 (week 2)	2
	3½	32 (week 1); 31 (week 2)	2
3 + 4	any distance	45 (week 3); 50 (week 4)	2
	4	36	2
	½ ; 4 × 1; ½	easy; 4 × 8½ ; easy	1
5 + 6	any distance	45 + 55 (week 5); 40 + 60 (week 6)	2
	5	47 (week 5); 46 (week 6)	2
7 + 8	any distance	40 + 60 (week 7); 40 + 65 (week 8)	2
	5	45	1
	1; 10 × 30 sec fast + 60 sec slow; 1	easy; fast; easy jog	1

continued

Weeks	Distance (miles)	Duration/pace (min)	Frequency per week
9 + 10	any distance	45 + 70	2
	1 ; 5 × 1	easy; fast	2
11 + 12	any distance	40 + 75	2
	5 + 6	easy + steady	2
13 + 14	any distance	40 + 80 (week 13); 85 (week 14)	2
	5 with 10 fast bursts	any	2
15 + 16	any distance	45 + 90 (week 15); 45 + 95 (week 16)	2
	1; 6 × 1; ½	easy; fast; easy	2
17 + 18	any distance	45 + 100 (week 17); 40 + 105 (week 18)	2
	1; 10 × 30-sec hills; 1	easy; fast; easy	2
19 + 20	any distance	50 + 110 (week 19); 40 + 115 (week 20)	2
	1; 6 × 1, 1	easy; fast; easy	2
21 + 22	any distance	45 + 120 (week 21); 40 + 125 (week 22)	2
	2; 4; 1	20 easy; 43 fast; 10 easy	2
23 + 24	any distance	50 + 130 (week 23); 45 + 135 (week 24)	2
	7	65 including 12-15 fast bursts	2

After week 24, here's what you should do in the remaining 2 weeks:

- Train on the same number of days per week, but gradually cut down the distances.
- Cut out the LSD runs of over 1 hour; keep up the steady runs over 4-6 miles.
- Do plenty of stretching.
- In the last 3-4 days focus on your eating: take in lots of carbohydrate and fluids. You may find it hard to eat large amounts of pasta, rice and bread as your appetite may have decreased with the decrease in training, but it is very important to do so as you want your body's carbohydrate stores completely full at the start of the marathon.

Gearing down

If aiming to run a marathon in 4½ hours seems a little too ambitious and you just want to finish it in any time, you can still follow the same programme but with these changes:

- Add about 2 minutes to the timed runs.
- Cut 10-15 minutes off the long runs.
- You could also drop 1 day of training per week.

Gearing up

If you have already completed a marathon in under 4½ hours and would like to go for a faster time, follow the same basic schedule, but push yourself a little harder:

- Add an extra ½-1 mile on the timed runs.
- Add an extra 10-15 minutes on the LSD runs.

Or

- Add an extra day of training to every second week.

Confidence booster

This programme doesn't mention any races, but it's a good idea to add in some 5- or 10-mile races and half-marathons in the last 3 months. This will get you used to road races and also add a bit of variety to your preparation. If you feel up to it, there are a few unusual distance races over 15 and 20 miles. It's a great confidence booster to know you can cover these distances before you tackle the full marathon distance.

SWIMMING

WHY SWIM?

Swimming is a great activity for developing aerobic fitness. It uses more muscles than most other popular sports, such as running or cycling, and is useful for developing your flexibility. This is due to the full range of movement that your arms go through during the stroke.

Because of the support of the water you can get a good workout in a non-weight-bearing activity, so there is less stress on your joints, which is important if you have any knee or ankle problems, or if you are overweight. Swimming, however, requires moderate skill to perform the strokes effectively, so you need to take lessons and practise to develop a good, efficient swimming style. Only then can you really use swimming as fitness training.

WHAT KIND OF SWIMMING IS FOR YOU?

If you are training for another sport and want to take a break or give your legs a rest, then swimming is ideal. But if you decide to progress with your swimming training and would like to compete, you will find there is quite a large gap between the serious recreational swimmer and the competitive swimmer. Unlike running, swimming lacks the all-comers 'fun run' element. But there are a number of events called 'duathlons' or 'biathlons', some combining swimming with cycling or running, and they are open to anyone. These can be great fun to take part in but you will need extra time to train for 2 sports rather than 1.

Recreational swimming

Recreational swimming is mainly aerobic in nature, as are any competitive distances over 200 m.

Competitive swimming

Swimming races range from 50 m up to 1500 m, using 1 stroke or a combination of all 4 strokes – known as a medley. The 4 swimming strokes are:

- 2 symmetrical – breaststroke and butterfly
- 2 asymmetrical – backstroke and front crawl.

Competitive training schedules for top swimmers are very arduous and time consuming, with many swimmers training 3 times per day.

- In the shorter events, the winner is the swimmer with the fastest reaction time at the start, the best technique in turning and touching at the finish and, of course, the fastest speed in the water.
- In the longer distances, these reaction times are less important than your actual swimming efficiency and aerobic fitness.

HOW THE WATER AFFECTS YOU

1. Your heart rate will be lower during swimming than in land-based sports due to the buoyancy effect of the water.
2. You lose heat more quickly when swimming. The layer of fat just underneath the skin acts as a protective layer to insulate against the cold. Very lean swimmers, therefore, may have problems in cold water.

Ideal water temperatures

- for learners about 30°C
- for recreational swimmers 28-30°C
- for competitive swimmers 25-27°C.

MUSCLES FOR SWIMMING

You use mainly your arms, plus other muscle groups depending on your stroke and your leg-kick pattern. In the front crawl you use 30-44 individual muscles. Good swimmers also use their trunk muscles (mainly abdominals) to keep a streamlined posture. Although it appears that the arms and shoulders generate most of the force in front crawl, better swimmers have a pronounced input from the trunk and the gluteus (backside). Top swimmers tend to use their trunk, pelvis and leg muscles properly (which also encourages correct swimming technique). Muscle strength is also important in swimming for the push-off from the tumble turn.

RISKS

Injuries in swimming are not too common and tend to be around the shoulder joint, especially if you do a lot of backstroke and front crawl, as both strokes push the shoulder to the limits of its range of motion.

ENERGY TO SWIM

Front crawl is the most economical stroke. It uses about 71% of the energy of backstroke. Not surprisingly, butterfly is the most demanding. Recreational swimmers use more energy in doing front crawl than treading water, whereas in the good swimmer the reverse is the case. A man of average weight would expect to burn up about 12 kilocalories per minute in butterfly, compared to 10 kilocalories per minute in front crawl. The average man would burn up about 200-240 kilocalories in 20 minutes of continuous swimming, regardless of stroke, and a woman would burn between 160-200 kilocalories in the same period.

> Did you know that you use up more energy doing the leg kick alone than doing either arms only or the whole stroke in either butterfly or breaststroke?

SWIMMER PROFILE

Anyone of any shape, age and size can swim. But your body shape (limb length, frame size, body-fat distribution), your muscular strength and endurance and your biomechanical ability will all affect your ability.

The good news for recreational swimmers is that a little extra fat helps your buoyancy and makes it easier for you to stay afloat. Competitive swimmers, on the other hand, tend to be tall and muscular with broad shoulders. Height can be an advantage in giving you a longer stroke and pipping your opponent at the finish. Average heights of Olympic swimmers are 181-191 cm and weights 70-80 kg. Although they are lean, swimmers carry a little more body fat than some other sports players such as runners or gymnasts, with levels of around 7% for top men and 19% for top women. It is very difficult to test the lung capacity of swimmers in the water and some are tested out of the water on specially adapted swim benches rigged up to a pulley system. Good swimmers have maximum oxygen-uptake levels of about 70 ml/kg/min (men) and 60 ml/kg/min (women). As you would expect, swimming training places high demands on your aerobic capacity.

ENTRY-LEVEL TRAINING

It is easy to get the impression that many competitive swimmers do no training other than swimming. This is not the case, as swimmers need to augment their swimming with additional strength training, and flexibility and shoulder-stability work. When you start training you should vary the stroke you use. Your weeks 1-3 could look as follows:

Week 1	*Stroke*	*Time/distance*	*Rest breaks*
Mon	front crawl	5-10 lengths	30 sec every 4 lengths
Tues	sidestroke	2 lengths each side	nil
Wed	rest day		
Thurs	optional day; repeat day 2 (i.e. Tuesday)		
Fri	front crawl	20 lengths	1 min every 5 lengths
Sat	rest day		
Sun	optional day; rest or repeat day 1 (i.e. Monday)		
Week 2			
Mon	1 of breaststroke 1 of front crawl	2 lengths of each for 10 min	2 min every 4 lengths
Tues	front crawl	10-30 lengths	30 sec every 8-10 lengths
Wed	rest day		
Thurs	rest day		
Fri	backstroke or breaststroke	6 lengths of each	1 min every 4 lengths
Sat	rest day		
Sun	rest day		
Week 3			
Mon	rest day		
Tues	as for Mon week 2		
Wed	rest day		
Thurs	as for Fri week 2		
Fri	your choice	5-10 min	2 min at 6-min mark
Sat	rest day		
Sun	rest day		

Aim to decrease the amount of rest between bouts of work so that, ultimately, you can complete your sessions without any rest at all. Try to include the more complex butterfly stroke. Once you have achieved all of this, not only will you be in good shape, but you may want to use some of the various towing hand paddles and flotation devices available which enable you to use legs only and arms only. Complete additional weight training and the rotator-cuff programme (page 164) 2-3 times per week on alternate days.

TRANSITION GOALS

If you are thinking about moving on to serious, competitive swimming training, ensure you can answer yes to the following questions:

1. Are you proficient in all swimming strokes?
2. Can you complete the entire entry-level swim programme, and each session, without rest breaks?
3. Are you consuming at least 2000-2500 calories per day, of which 70% are complex carbohydrates?
4. Do you have swimming goggles, ear plugs and other equipment specified by your club?
5. Have you spoken to a qualified swimming coach or expert at a swimming club?
6. Have you completed 6-8 weeks of strength training? That is, a minimum of 20 weight-training and 20 rotator-cuff programmes?
7. Are you injury free, especially in the shoulder and upper-limb area?

ADVANCED-LEVEL TRAINING

At competitive levels training is very demanding. Most swimmers will complete at least 1 major session per day; many will complete 2 or even 3 sessions. As all competitive swimmers will have the input of a coach, there is little point in covering what you should complete in a session, especially considering the variety of disciplines and distances available to race in. What remains most important is your supplementary programme. Muscle imbalances are common in swimmers who only swim. Such imbalances, in which one group of muscles is far stronger than another (or more flexible), lead to injuries and overuse syndromes.

"3

Rotator cuff and flexibility

Most training, regardless of your preferred stroke, should involve all of the major strokes such as front crawl, and backstroke in particular. Doing a variety of strokes will help to maintain muscle balance, but it is still crucial for you to complete the rotator-cuff programme. You should also emphasize those areas of the cuff which do the least work.

If you are predominantly a front-crawl swimmer, the muscles at the front of the cuff and the front shoulder and chest muscles become especially strong. Those muscles at the rear of the cuff and the back of the shoulder are weaker. You should therefore complete 25-30% more rotator-cuff work. You need to complete those exercises which draw the arm away from the body and slightly backwards (including rotation of the upper arm away from the body).

Base strength training

Base strength training is the key to becoming a far better swimmer. Improving your strength will increase your power through the water. Using your legs correctly and improving the power in your legs will add some considerable speed to your stroke. Obviously, improving upper-body strength will lead to greater power in your arms.

8-week rotation of training

Be sure to rest during week 9, to allow your body to recover before repeating the cycle. If you don't have time to do both swimming training and supplementary training, do a little of each rather than cut out one area entirely. For all exercises, see Chapter 5, page 48.

Weeks	Emphasis/ frequency per week	Notes
1+2	muscle endurance/ 2	use multi-gym equipment; complete the entry-level 'core' strength programme: 3 sets of 40 repetitions of each exercise in circuit manner
3+4	strength/3	complete the advanced-level 'core' strength programme: 7-9 repetitions, 2 sets of each exercise; complete all sets in 1 exercise before moving on

continued

Weeks	Emphasis/ frequency per week	Notes
5+6	power/2	complete 4 sets of 3 repetitions of the following exercises, resting for 4 min between sets: dead lifts, free-weight bench, lateral pull down
7+8	strength/2	repeat weeks 3 and 4

SKIING

The word 'ski' is Norwegian in origin, and skiing is the most popular sport in Scandinavia. About 50% of Swedish people between the ages of 18 and 70 years ski regularly. Unlike the rest of us, who mainly concentrate on 'downhill' skiing, Scandinavians go in for 'cross-country' skiing. Note that injuries are almost threefold in downhill skiing in comparison to its cross-country cousin.

What type of skier are you?

Most skiers ski once a year, probably for a week, and always promise themselves that, next year, they will spend more time making sure they are fit. Are you more experienced than this? If so, you probably learnt to ski at an early age and now spend some weeks skiing every year, looking for the most difficult off-piste runs. More keen still? In that case, you may even spend seasons as a ski instructor. Finally, you may be a competitive skier at national level. Your main events are downhill, special slalom and giant slalom.

HOW DEMANDING IS SKIING?

Heart rate

Level	Heart rate
recreational	about 140-160 bpm on your runs, depending on the type of course
more experienced	about 160-170 bpm on the downhills

Your heart rate will drop right down as you recover in the ski lift, ready for the next run. This is just as well, as it would be very difficult to sustain this level of intensity for the length of time most of you spend on the slopes. This heart rate would equate to about 40-50% of your maximum aerobic capacity over the course of a day's skiing, which appears quite low but is higher in more experienced skiers. But remember, it is because of the moderate intensity that you can continue skiing on and off all day.

Aerobic and anaerobic systems

Skiing places high demands on the aerobic system at all levels, events such as the giant slalom being the most demanding and requiring a good anaerobic system too. The amount of energy contributed from the anaerobic energy system increases as your standard improves. Good performance in competitive skiing demands about 50% endurance, 30% anaerobic power and 20% flexibility/agility. You should use these figures as a guide when preparing for skiing at any level.

ENERGY

Skiing can be quite demanding on your body's energy stores, particularly as you have to stay on the slopes for several hours. At the end of each day your muscles' carbohydrate stores (glycogen) will be almost completely empty and it is important that you replenish these for the next day's skiing. If you don't, you will find that you get tired easily after about 4 days. The typical energy use during skiing is about 360 kilocalories per hour in women and about 480 kilocalories per hour in men.

> Don't forget that you are more likely to sustain an injury when fatigued. It is unwise to ski if you are prone to knee problems.

SKIER PROFILE

Recreational skiers

There is no ideal body type or shape for the recreational skier. However, to prepare for and enjoy skiing at any level you need to develop a good aerobic capacity, good leg strength and flexibility. It is also important to eat a high-carbohydrate diet while skiing and to pace yourself over the first few days.

Competitive skiers

Competitive skiers tend to be small and lean with well-developed muscles, and have body-fat levels of about 11-12% (men), 18-20% (women). Modest stature is important as shorter legs lower the centre of gravity and improve balance when turning. Competitive skiers also have a high aerobic capacity with VO_2 max levels of 70 ml/kg/min in men and 58 ml/kg/min in women. Cross-country competitive skiers have even higher levels, as high as 80 ml/kg/min (men) and 70 ml/kg/min (women). Indeed, cross-country skiers are among the fittest of sportspeople. Due to the particular physical demands of skiing, competitive skiers develop above-average dynamic and iso-metric leg strength, especially in the quadriceps, and superior grip strength.

Please note: most injuries occur in the afternoon of the first or second day of a skiing holiday.

ENTRY-LEVEL TRAINING

So you want to ski? Or maybe you already do but have never really got fit for skiing? With a little regular effort you need never feel that post-ski soreness again. At the very least, you can significantly reduce it. You need 3 basic types of fitness to get into skiing or to enjoy your week's skiing to the full:

- flexibility
- muscle strength
- good aerobic capacity.

Flexibility

Before you begin a training session, remember to complete the flexibility (stretching) exercises suggested in Chapter 6. Then complete those on page 192, which are specific to skiing movement.

Remember to complete these exercises after training and before and after skiing.

Stretches for flexibility

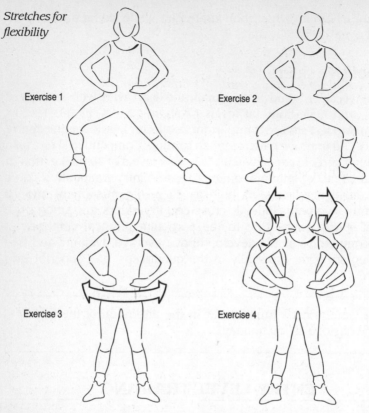

Hold each stretch for 15-20 seconds and complete 4 each side (exercises 1 and 2). You should feel the stretch at the inner thigh. When doing the rotation and bending movements (exercises 3 and 4) be careful to work within your limits. These are gentle mobility movements and should be performed for 30 seconds each. Do not move with great speed and use a comfortable range of movement.

Muscular-strength and endurance training

Follow the circuit below and bear in mind that any aerobic work you do which uses your legs will also improve the endurance in those muscles. You should use a gym for the 4-5 weeks leading up to your skiing, concentrating on working up to very high repetitions and moving through the circuit 4-6 times.

Complete 25-35 repetitions for all the following exercises (except the abdominal crunches). Complete 15 repetitions when doing the abdominal crunches. Go through this whole circuit 2-6 times.

1. Leg press, using 1 leg at a time. Swap legs after completing each set.
2. Bench press.
3. Lunges with light dumbbells. Bend the front leg no more than 90 degrees when lunging forward.
4. Dumbbell shoulder press with light dumbbells.
5. Lateral pull down behind the neck.
6. Half squats with moderately heavy dumbbells.
7. Abdominal crunches.

Aerobic conditioning

Do you want to ski for a day without undue fatigue? Would you like to complete those long runs with style? The aerobic programme suggested here will also improve muscle endurance in your legs. Try to train 3-4 times a week.

Day 1
Light jogging or running. Vary the terrain where possible, for example running on a golf course, beach, track, etc. Train for 15-30 minutes as you begin to improve.

Day 2
Step class or stepping machine (this is available at most gyms and involves a continuous stepping movement on raised steps with a set resistance). If you join a class (you may even find a ski-conditioning class) you will need to work for about 45 minutes. If you use the step machine, work out for 20-30 minutes on a varied-terrain (often known as a random or interval) programme.

Day 3
Cycle, use the rowing machine or jog/run again. If cycling, work for 30-40 minutes, if rowing work for 20 minutes, and if jogging/running work for 25-30 minutes. Remember, if you have difficulty jogging for the whole time you can alternate between jogging/running and walking, but keep moving!

The more weeks of training you can complete before you ski the more enjoyable your time on the slopes will be. But, most importantly, you will also reduce the risk of slight sprains and strains. Do a minimum of 4 weeks' training and try and go up to 8 weeks.

Your training week

This is the ideal and includes the muscle-endurance circuit. So, on some days you will complete both on the same day.

Mon	muscle-endurance circuit; day 1 aerobic programme
Tues	rest
Wed	day 2 aerobic programme
Thurs	muscle-endurance circuit
Fri	day 3 aerobic programme
Sat	repeat day 3 aerobic programme; muscle-endurance circuit
Sun	rest

TRANSITION GOALS

You should have completed the entry-level programme successfully before you start weeks 1-4 of the advanced-level programme.

ADVANCED-LEVEL TRAINING

At competitive level, or for those of you who plan a prolonged skiing holiday (season), the physical demands are staggering. At this level you should be able to ski for 2-3 hours at a time. Leg-muscle endurance, explosive power when turning and the ability to recover quickly are now very desirable.

Aerobic conditioning

You must complete the warm-up/cool-down and stretching exercises described in the entry-level training programme.

Weeks 1-4
Complete 4 aerobic sessions per week. Rotate between running (soft surfaces), rowing machine, step machine, cycling and swimming. Work for 30-50 minutes at 75% of MHR.

Weeks 5-8
Complete 2 interval sessions and continue with 2 additional continuous aerobic sessions, following the format for weeks 1-4.

Interval training session 1: Use the step machine, cycle or row. Work at 85-90% of MHR for 1 minute then drop the level of intensity to 50-60% MHR for 2 minutes. This is 1 repetition. Complete 2 sets (6 repetitions in each set) with 5 minutes' light work (40% MHR) between sets.

Interval training session 2: Run for this session, either on an outdoor hard or soft surface, or on a treadmill. Ensure you do this only if your knees, hips and ankles are injury free. If they are not, use the modes suggested in session 1. Now make the intervals 1 minute 'on' and 1 minute 'off'. Again, complete 6 repetitions per set and do 2 sets.

Training for more than 8 weeks
If you have the time available to train over and above the 8-week mark, your priority should be not to add more sessions but to increase the intensity of the work. Increase to 2 minutes 'on' and 1 minute 'off'. Your continuous training should stay as suggested.

Strength, endurance and power training

The following progressions result in an improved strength base. With this strength you will also gain improved endurance, although this is more apparent in later weeks. Power, in the form of plyometric work, is introduced to give that added explosiveness if you are competing.

Weeks 1-4

Session 1: Do the pre-exhaustion training programme suggested in Chapter 5 (page 53). Remember to work to failure. Complete 7-9 repetitions for each exercise. Complete 3 sets of each exercise before moving on to the next exercise.

Sessions 2 and 3: As session 1.

Weeks 5-8

Session 1: As above for session 1.

Session 2: Use the pre-exhaustion training programme but complete 50-60 repetitions in each set and work through as a circuit, moving from one exercise to the next. Complete 4-5 circuits per session.

Session 3: Complete the acceleration programme in Chapter 7 using the programme set out for weeks 3 and 4 in the advanced-level programme (page 75). Complete this work only if you are injury free. Begin at half the recommended repetitions and sets and gradually build up.

Your overall training plan should look similar to this:

Weeks 1-4	
Mon	continuous aerobic and strength (session 1)
Tues	rest
Wed	as for Monday
Thurs	continuous aerobic
Fri	as for Monday
Sat	rest
Sun	rest

Weeks 5-8	
Mon	continuous aerobic and strength (session 1)
Tues	interval aerobic (session 1)
Wed	rest
Thurs	power training (session 3), then continuous aerobic training (session 1)
Fri	interval training (session 2)
Sat	muscle-rest endurance training (session 2)
Sun	rest

After 8 weeks of training at this intensity it is important to have a very light week. Complete just 2 aerobic sessions (continuous). Thereafter, time and actual skiing permitting, repeat the cycle for weeks 5-8.

SNOW BOARDING

Snow boarding is an off-shoot of skiing that has very similar fitness demands. Little research is available which examines the exact demands of snow boarding but there are several areas that need special attention for your day to be a success.

The program set out for the skier is largely what the boarder also requires and is solid preparation for the sport (see pages 189-96). However the snow boarder has the unique situation of having both feet fixed (much like a surfer or skate boarder) and as a consequence needs excellent abdominal strength and stability to control the board. For this reason, incorporating core stability is important. Routines based on an exercise ball (often referred to as a Swiss ball) are an excellent way to improved abdominal control. A wide variety of exercises exist and examples are usually provided with the ball which can be purchased at a sports equipment outlet.

Balance is more difficult for the snowboarder than the skier. Changes in terrain are harder to compensate for when your feet are together, and they place high demands on knee, ankle and hip joint proprioception – the ability for you to react instantly to a loss of balance and avoid falling. The use of a wobble board or balance pad is an excellent way to improve balance, particularly if you can do the exercises with your eyes closed. Placing your board on top of the wobble board or pad is even more specific, with the key being to retain your balance on an unstable platform.

Finally, you will find the addition of a little extra strength to be an advantage. Getting up from a fall demands not only technique but also a fair amount of leg and often upper body strength to initiate the movement of getting up, particularly off-piste. Therefore an extra 4 weeks of strength training added to the skiing program would be well advised, resulting in an 8 to 12 week preparation period with the extra strength work incorporated into the start of you training.

GOLF

Golf is a game for people of all shapes, sizes and abilities and is extremely popular throughout the world. The handicap system allows you to play a competitive game against a more (or less) experienced player. If you are new to the game your handicap starts at 26 (men) and 36 (women). Men have a lower handicap as, in theory, they should be able to get around in fewer shots than women. The handicap lowers with improvement – you have less chance of compensating for your bad shots – so it becomes more of a challenge to play to your handicap. At professional level no allowance is made for handicap so no one has an advantage.

Golf can be as competitive as you want it to be – it can be you against the course or, if you opt for match play, it's you against your opponent. It can also be a very sociable game. With club draws you never know who you will end up playing against.

Depending on the course, golf can be played all year round. On European parkland courses it tends to be more popular from spring through to autumn. A course can be from 6 to 13 km, but 7 km is average for 18 holes. But it is a lot further if you are walking from one side of the fairway to the other much of the time. Courses can be flat or on the side of a mountain, with any amount of natural and placed hazards.

Training and conditioning were neglected in golf until the 1960s when Gary Player made players aware that off-season fitness training could improve their game. These days most professional golfers train seriously.

Why should you train?

1. By doing specific strengthening and conditioning your performance will improve.
2. It will help to reduce the risk of injury.

HOW DEMANDING IS GOLF?

Golf is a relatively gentle sport which requires only moderate aerobic capacity and muscle endurance. It is sometimes considered a 'soft' game in terms of intensity or how strenuous it is, but when playing an

198

average game of golf, whether pulling a caddie car or carrying your clubs, you would be exercising at about 35-41% of your maximum aerobic capacity at a heart rate between 90 and 120 beats per minute. As this is below the level (60-80% VO_2 max) usually recommended to train the heart and lungs, golf is not the best sport to choose to get you fit. However, the low intensity encourages your body to burn more fat as a fuel and uses up between 4 and 6 kilocalories per minute. In a 4-hour game you could burn up about 1200 kilocalories, which is no mean feat. Golf may not get you fit, but proper training for golf should improve strength and flexibility and burn up some calories in the process.

Energy and muscles

Golf is very demanding on many muscle groups in terms of strength and flexibility. Your legs need to be strong enough to walk around the course at a reasonable pace and to get power behind shots. How fast and how far you can hit the ball is determined by the club head and by the speed at which you swing your arms in the forward swing. If you are a right-handed golfer your left arm determines how far you can hit the ball. Your upper-back muscles, the latissimus dorsi, do the work during this action. These are the muscles that you use doing a lateral pull down or a chin-up exercise on a resistance machine in the gym. The shoulders, particularly the rotator cuff, need to have a good range of motion – without muscle tension, which is detrimental to the swing. You also use your forearm in the golfing action. Since back injuries and lower-back strain are hazards for regular golfers, strong abdominal muscles are important to support your back. Flexibility of the rotator cuff and hips (for trunk rotation) is also a key element in golf.

> Even if you do none of the other training recommended in this section, at least do the flexibility exercise for the rotator cuff and hips. You will notice an improvement in your game through this exercise alone.

PLAYER PROFILE

There is no ideal height or weight for golf, although shorter players may find it more difficult to get the same power behind their shots as taller players. In fitness terms, golfers are a little above the general population average for VO$_2$ max, with good, young male club players reaching about 45-50 ml/kg/min. Broadly speaking, your fitness tends to increase as your handicap goes down. However, this is not necessarily true for professional female golfers, who have VO$_2$ max levels no higher than average (34 ml/kg/min) and body-fat levels of about 24% (the same as a normal, inactive person).

TRAINING FOR GOLF

Whether you are a once-a-fortnight fair-weather golfer or a low-handicap club player, your game will certainly benefit from some planned training to improve your flexibility, strength and general aerobic fitness. You need:

- flexibility, especially in the rotation of the spine and hips
- suppleness in your shoulder, back and groin
- forearm strength
- grip strength.

Good golfers have excellent hand-grip strength, particularly in the left hand (if you are right-handed). Good strength in the forearms, and back and shoulder flexibility will help you hit faster and hence further.

If you improve your aerobic capacity you will be able to cover the distances between holes more easily. Aerobic fitness has also been shown to help concentration. As fatigue sets in, concentration can falter and mistakes can be made. This also applies to muscle endurance – as muscles become fatigued, errors tend to occur.

ENTRY-LEVEL TRAINING

At this level, you need only supplement your play with 2 or possibly 3 training sessions a week. Your training week could look as follows (add in another circuit or aerobic day if you have the time):

Mon	aerobic 1
Tue	circuit 1
Wed	rest
Thurs	aerobic 2
Fri	circuit 2
Sat	rest
Sun	rest

Aerobic 1 and 2

You can swim (great for improving shoulder mobility), cycle or jog. Work at 60-70% of your maximum heart rate. Make the training last for 15-20 minutes and slowly build on this until you can work for 30-40 minutes. You can rest from time to time, but endeavour to work continually over this period.

Circuits 1 and 2

Complete the entry-level programmes in Chapter 5 (page 52).

Circuit 1: In your first session, complete 30-35 repetitions of each exercise before moving on to the next. Complete the circuit 3-5 times.

Circuit 2: Repeat using a heavier weight and complete 10 repetitions of the exercise. Complete the circuit 2-3 times only.

Don't worry if you do not have access to weight-training equipment. Try the following circuit instead of circuits 1 and 2.

Exercise	Repetitions
half squat	40-50
press-ups	15-30
dips	10-30
lunges	20-40 total
twist to touch the wall	20 each side
crunch sit-ups	20-40
alternate arm punches	20-40 each side

- Complete the number of repetitions you feel comfortable with within the range suggested.
- Complete the circuit 3-7 times.
- Aim to complete the circuit, without resting, at a comfortable pace.
- You can rest as you need to when you are working at between 60% and 75% of your maximum.

Flexibility

As golf requires a good deal of rotation in the spine, being more flexible will help your swing as well as allowing you to increase the power and control of your shots. If you are taking up the game later in life, complete the core exercises in Chapter 6 (page 59).

In addition, all players should complete the following exercises:

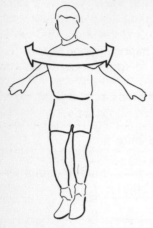

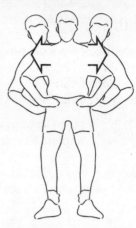

1. Side twists, 20 to each side.   2. Side bends, 20 to each side.

3. Double-club swing: take 2 irons and gently swing a full swing. Do this 10 times.

The majority of golfers experience some tightness in the lower back from time to time. Although the upper back and neck are both well designed for rotation, the lower back is not. Your lower back must be supple to ensure that *all* of the spine takes the stress of the swing. Do the stretches for the back as recommended in Chapter 6.

Back-stretching exercises

1. *Knees to chest*: Lying on your back, pull the knees into the chest and hold for 1-2 seconds. Complete 10-15 times.

2. *Opposite knee to shoulder*: Lying on your back, pull one knee up and over towards the opposite shoulder. Alternate between the left and right, and complete 10 each side.

3. *Back extensions*: Lying on your front, keep your hips on the ground – this is important. Tighten your gluteal (buttock) muscles and push

up, arching your back. Only lift 15-20 cm off the floor – your arms don't necessarily need to straighten. Hold each extension for 2 seconds. Complete 10-20 times.

ADVANCED-LEVEL TRAINING

If you are a serious golfer, one who plays at least once a week, or indeed on a semi-professional level, your game will benefit considerably from a physical-fitness regime. At an advanced level, 18-36 holes in a day (that's 4-8 hours of high concentration) is not uncommon. High aerobic levels, good strength and good spinal rotation become ever more important.

If you play 2 rounds per week, your programme may look as follows:

Mon	round 1 then weights
Tues	aerobic
Wed	round 2 then weights
Thurs	aerobic
Fri	rest
Sat	competition
Sun	rest or competition

Strength training

Complete the pre-exhaustion training programme detailed in Chapter 5 (page 53). Add weeks 8-12 at repetitions of 7-9 per set for each exercise (except abdominal curls). Rest from all training in the 7th or 13th week before repeating the cycle. Then complete the following exercises at the end of your programme.

Forearm curls

Curls improve the strength endurance of the muscles which support the elbow, a common area for injury ('golfer's elbow').

1. Rest your forearms on a bench, palms up, and, using a weight (either barbell or dumbbells), curl the wrists up.
2. Slowly curl them down.
3. Complete 10-12 repetitions in a set and complete 2-3 sets.

Flexibility

1. Complete the stretches and mobility exercises detailed in the entry-level section, but double the repetitions. Your flexibility is vital to your swing and to prevent injuries, especially chronic ones which build up over a long period. Golfer's elbow can be especially insidious and can keep you out of the game for some time.

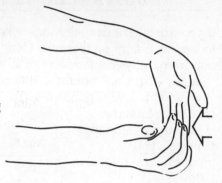

2. In addition to the strength-training exercises described above, complete the following stretch to help prevent injury.

Aerobic programme

Aim to improve your overall stamina level and your concentration. Train twice a week for the full 12 weeks before taking a rest week. Keep as much variety as possible in your programme.

Week	Session	Details
1	1	swim 15-20 min, mixing front crawl and backstroke; rest every 3 lengths
	2	cycle 20 min continuous at 65% MHR
2	3	step machine for 20 min on a random programme 70% MHR
	4	jogging 20 min at 60-75% MHR
3	5	swim mixed strokes for 30 min, resting every 4 lengths
	6	cycle 30 min, random programme at 80% MHR
4	7	step machine 30 min on a continuous programme; 80% MHR
	8	jogging 30 min at 50-60% MHR

continued

Week	Session	Details
5	9	as week 3
	10	as week 3
6	11	as week 4
	12	as week 4
7	13	swim 2 lengths as fast as possible, any stroke; rest for 3 min; repeat this cycle for 40 min
	14	as for session 13
8	15	step machine; 2 min at 80% MHR; then 2-3 min at 50% MHR; repeat cycle for 40 min
	16	as for session 15
9	17	cycle for 30 min continuously at 60% MHR
	18	jogging for 30 min at 50% MHR
10	19	repeat session 13
	20	repeat session 13
11	21	repeat session 15
	22	repeat session 1
12	23	repeat session 5
	24	repeat session 6

In subsequent rotations of this programme, try to increase all workouts by 5-10 minutes until each session is 40-50 minutes in duration.

CYCLING

Which type of cyclist are you?

1. You use it to get you comfortably from A to B.
2. It is your chosen form of exercise or training.

While cycling, you have to balance on an unstable 2-wheeled machine, simultaneously providing the force to move it forward and control your speed and direction. On an open, unobstructed flat surface without traffic you are no more likely to be injured than if you were walking or jogging. But the speed and close proximity to other cyclists in competitive races make cycling a very dangerous sport with a high risk of injury.

WHEN AND WHERE?

If you are a competitive or fun cyclist you will mainly be cycling between April and October. There are plenty of cycling clubs around catering for a wide range of abilities and many different cycle events to take part in. One of the tougher ones in England is the London to Brighton race (approximately 88.5 km). Quite a challenge even for the fittest! So, if you have taken up or plan to take up cycling and need new routes, some challenges or some company to cycle with, hunt out your local cycle club and see what they have to offer.

ENERGY AND MUSCLES

Cycling is very much a lower-body activity, using the quadriceps muscle, the gluteus muscle (the backside area at the top of the hamstring) and the hamstrings to complete the action of pedalling.

Competitive cycling

Whether on the track or the road, racing places extremely high demands on your physical capacity. Races range from a 200-m track sprint which might take less than 10 seconds up to the 5000-km (approximately) Tour de France which lasts 23 days. Most of the longer-distance races are on the road. A high aerobic capacity is required to cope with cycling continuously for a long time. However, to cope with hills, accelerations and occasional sprints, you also need a good anaerobic capacity. Track races over shorter distances are more demanding on your power and speed endurance. Whether on the road or the track, cycling requires you to exercise at a high percentage of your maximum aerobic capacity.

Recreational cycling

As your body weight is supported you need to cover about 3-5 times the distance you could achieve in the same time by jogging to use the same amount of calories. Initially, cycling can result in local muscle tiredness in your legs before your heart and lungs are adequately stressed. However, as you improve and adapt, cycling becomes more of a whole-body activity.

CYCLIST PROFILE

The good news is that it doesn't matter what shape or height you are. A smaller cyclist may have the advantage of a lower aerodynamic resistance, especially in windy conditions. But, if you are larger, you have a larger lung capacity and greater power for hill climbs and accelerations. Since your body weight is supported in cycling, even if you are not slim, you are not at a disadvantage provided the extra weight is muscle and not fat. A high muscle-to-fat ratio is a must for a good cyclist – again, particularly for those hill climbs, when power in the legs gives you a distinct advantage. Body fat in top-level cyclists is about 6-9% for men and about 12-15% for women, which is low and reflects the many hours cyclists spend in the saddle.

A high aerobic capacity is a must for success in competitive cycling, and some of the highest values recorded for maximal oxygen uptake are in top-level cyclists. Even those who race over the shorter track distance need to have a good aerobic capacity to cope with the very demanding training. Men have maximum VO_2 levels of 70-80 ml/kg/min and women are in the region of 60-70 ml/kg/min.

You must be able to exercise at a high percentage of your VO_2 max. Trained cyclists can often continue exercising up to and above 75-85% of the VO_2 max before reaching their anaerobic threshold.

What is a good cycling position?

If you are cycling outdoors, not in a gym, lean a little forward on the handlebars, or assume a semi-upright position rather than sitting straight up. This is more aerodynamic and will reduce wind resistance. There is no point in making it any harder than it has to be!

EQUIPMENT

Your choice of bike depends on your intended use. If you want a bike to cycle around town, and some roads are quite bumpy, then you may be better off with a mountain bike. This leaves you with the option of

going on trails and off-road rides. However, if you want to train seriously and have a go at a few races, then you need to consider getting
a racing bike, which is lighter and has lower wind resistance.

Which is the right-size bike for you?

The easiest way to determine the correct frame is to straddle the bike
at the top tube/bar. There should be about 2-3 cm between your
crotch and the tube/bar. A more accurate method involves measuring
your leg length. Measure from the top of your leg, at the hip, to your
heel in bare feet. You can gauge the right place by turning your foot in
and out to feel where the top of your leg bone is. Take this figure and
subtract 34 cm and this will be your correct frame size. The correct
seat height should allow you a very slight bend in the knee when the
pedal is in the down position.

Should you use toe straps, cleated shoes or normal pedals?

Toe clips are an advantage only for competitive cyclists. Using cleated
shoes delays fatigue in your quadriceps by spreading the workload.
Otherwise, normal pedals are fine.

Pedal speeds, measured as revolutions per minute (rpm), can
make a difference in terms of efficiency. Trained cyclists pedal
between 70 and 102 rpm, with their preferred speed of 90 rpm. It is
actually easier to pedal faster when you add resistance on a stationary
cycle or on a flat surface in a high gear. However, too high a pedal
speed increases your tendency to make extra body movements, which
makes you less efficient all round, so watch out for this.

ENTRY-LEVEL TRAINING

Flexibility

Cyclists are prone to tightness in their gluteal (buttock) and hamstring
muscles, as well as in their calves. The gluteal and hamstring muscles
have a direct effect on the back, and keeping these areas supple is crucial in protecting your back. You will also notice the bent-over position you assume on the bike: this 'forward flexion' position needs to
be counteracted through your flexibility programme. In addition to the

core flexibility programme outlined in Chapter 6, you should include the following exercises. Remember, you must do them *before* and, crucially, *after* you go out for a training ride.

Back extensions

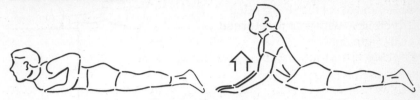

Lie flat on the ground, face down. Be sure to keep your hips on the ground at all times.

1. Arch your back as far as you can without causing discomfort.
2. Hold this for 2–3 seconds.
3. Do this 10 times, lowering yourself each time.
4. Repeat, but come up slightly towards the right.
5. Repeat again, but come up slightly towards the left.
6. Repeat 4 and 5, alternating sides each time, and do 10 of each.

Hamstring stretch

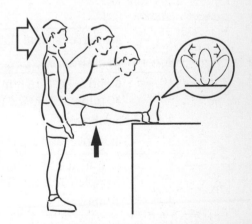

1. Complete the hamstring stretch shown.
2. Hold 2–3 repetitions with your foot straight.
3. Hold 2–3 repetitions with your foot turned out.
4. Hold 2–3 repetitions with your foot turned in. Remember: your leg should remain straight and so should your back. Lean forward at the hips.

> Do these exercises in conjunction with a general programme. Do not do them on their own as this would create muscle imbalance rather than help prevent it.

5. Repeat the hamstring stretch, but this time keep your leg very slightly bent. You will feel this stretch more in the belly of the (deep middle) muscle.
6. Repeat as for the straight-leg version – with your foot turned in, then out.

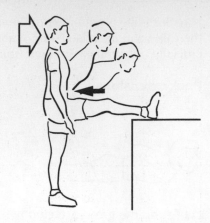

Training programme

If you want to join in any organized events, join a cycling club. You will find an enormous variety of events, and you will need an expert's help to prepare successfully for whichever one you choose. If, however, you wish to use cycling as a way to improve your aerobic fitness and lower-limb muscle tone, try the following programme:

Week	Session	Details
1	1	30-min easy ride, flat terrain, 50-70% MHR
	2	as above
2	1	5 min at 60%, 15 min at 75-80%, 5 min at 50%, 10 min at 75-80%, 5 min at 60%, 10 min at 75-80%
	2	as above
	3	as above; add 1-2 min to each block of work
3	1	10 min at 50%; 5 min at 70% then 5 min at 50%; complete this rotation for 40 min
	2	as above
4	1	45 min at 50-60%
	2	60 min at 60-70%
	3	75 min at 50%

continued

Week	Session	Details
5	1	10-15 min at 40-50%, then 2 min at 80-85% followed by 3-4 min at 40-50%; repeat this pattern for 10 min; cruise for 4-5 min and repeat the pattern for 45-75 min
	2	30 min at 50-60%
	3	as for session 1, week 5
6	1	as week 2
	2	as week 2
	3	as week 2

In week 7, have a rest week and emphasize your stretching. In subsequent repeats of this programme, aim to add in some hills and increase your workout periods to 90 minutes. If you are very keen, you can train for up to 120 minutes.

ADVANCED-LEVEL TRAINING

Much of your training will depend on your cycling work, your coach or your club. If you are doing sprint events, power training can really help. This type of exercise occurs within cycle training, usually via short, explosive sprints of 40-100 m, or hill sprints. So, if your event involves more than 1 cycling session per day, you will already be placing your legs under tremendous pressure, and extra work will be of little benefit. If, however, your work on the bike is only 1 session per day, you will get additional power through weight training.

If you are participating in long events you will gain little from weight training (unless you have a muscular imbalance) as even the highest repetition training will not mimic the many thousands of leg-muscle contractions you already complete in a training ride or event.

Remember, always complete a thorough warm-up and stretch before training. At advanced levels you need flexibility far more than at entry level, as good free movement = efficiency. If you are flexible, you can easily maintain an aerodynamic body position and freedom of movement in your legs.

Explosive movements will improve with high-intensity, low-repetition (heavy-weight) training. Complete the core advanced-training programme in Chapter 5 (page 48), making the following adjustments:

1. Complete 4-6 sets of 1-3 repetitions in the half squat.
2. Complete 4-6 sets of 10-12 repetitions per set in the hamstring curl.
3. Complete only 1-2 sets of the upper-body exercises, completing only 7-9 repetitions of each exercise.
4. Complete the following 2 additional exercises for the upper and mid-back:

Dumbbell flys reverse

This exercise helps to prevent rounded shoulders and neck problems.

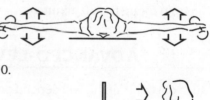

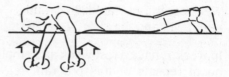

1. Lie on a bench face down.
2. Use reasonably heavy dumbbells.
3. Lift your arms up (in a 'flying' action).
4. At the top of the movement, hold the position for a count of 10.
5. Lower the weights slowly.

Pectoral (chest) stretch

This exercise helps to maintain good posture.

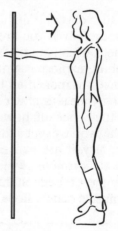

1. Place your straight arm behind a pole.
2. Move your body in the opposite direction until a stretch is felt in your chest.

Resistance training

Do this 2-3 times per week, on alternate days, depending on your cycling workload. Just a little training will improve your posture on the bike, help prevent upper-, lower-back and neck problems, and add additional power to the sprint events. Complete the base strength programme for the first 8 weeks (advanced level), then move on to the muscle endurance programme (repetitions over 40 per set) for the following 6 weeks. Rest for 1 week then repeat this cycle.

GROUP EXERCISE AND STUDIO CLASSES

Exercise or dance routines performed to music have been extremely popular for many years and can offer an enjoyable and motivating way to exercise. Classes and routines can be adapted to any skill or fitness level and the lack of competition allows individuals to work at their own pace The range and choice of classes continues to develop and expand and provide a great alternative to traditional outdoor sports.

AEROBICS AND ITS VARIATIONS

Since the aerobics boom in the 1980s, aerobics as an umbrella term now covers a multitude of different class choices with a variety of different names. Most tend to fall into one of these exercise types:

- high- and low-impact aerobics
- step
- dance beat – cardio funk/hip hop
- water-based – aqua
- body toning/sculpting/conditioning

All can be a great way of adding variety to your workout. The amount of benefit you get is entirely up to you and how hard you push yourself. How strenuous you find a class is determined on your fitness level, shape and weight, as well as by the technical difficulty in terms of routines or choreography.

BENEFITS AND RISKS

The benefits include:

- attaining good, overall aerobic fitness
- good off-season exercise.

There has been concern about injuries, particularly those associated with high-impact aerobics or step aerobics. Common types of injury include:

- shin splints
- stress fractures
- tendon problems
- overuse problems in the knees and lower back.

The shoes you wear and the type of floor in the class are often the cause.

Anyone with a history of knee injuries or problems should be careful with any type of aerobics exercise as classes often include movements with increased flexion of the knee. Discuss your knee problem with the instructor, who will advise you which movements to avoid or to adapt. Also, it is always tempting to do too much, partly because you see others 'keeping up' and partly because there are so many enticing classes. But doing too much is hazardous if you are unfit or new to exercise.

ENERGY AND MUSCLES

Aerobics is not effective in increasing strength or power. But some classes include muscle-conditioning exercises which help tone up your muscles. Any change in body shape will occur through a loss of body fat, not bigger muscles.

If you compare the energy used in a high-intensity/high-impact aerobics class with that used in a low-intensity/low-impact class you'll notice a substantial difference in the average heart rate:

	Low	High	Low impact/ high intensity
heart rate	130 bpm	174 bpm	164 bpm
% of maximum capacity	37%	70-78%	80-85%
kcals	5 per min	10 per min	8 per min

Low impact, high intensity

A low-intensity class (see below) does little for your aerobic fitness. But low-impact/high-intensity classes are ideal for improving fitness as they include plenty of arms-above-shoulders movements and leg kicks, which use the same beat as a high-impact class. How much energy you use depends very much on:

- type of music (beats per minute)
- muscle movements
- type of impact
- type and duration of the warm-up and cool-down.

High or low impact?

Low-impact classes are particularly useful for a beginner if you are overweight, pregnant, or have knee or lower-back trouble. With any high-impact activity, the impact of your body landing on the ground can be equivalent to 7 times your body weight. This sends tiny shock waves through your joints, from your ankle to your hip and lower back. Low-impact aerobics avoids this as 1 foot must be in contact with the ground at all times. To increase the intensity, upper-body movements are accentuated.

If you are very fit you may find it difficult to raise your heart rate into the target zone when keeping a foot on the ground. However, a good instructor can put together an effective low-impact class with some clever arm movements.

THE LOW-DOWN ON AEROBICS CLASSES

Aerobics is typically a combination of high- and/or low-impact moves in set choreographed patterns, using several known steps and moves, interspersed with the instructor's own style. These classes can be useful for developing a good basic level of fitness and conditioning.

Dance beat aerobics usually involves more choreographed routines incorporating a range of dance moves and up-beat music. Good co-ordination and rhythm are useful. The tempo of the music and moves can keep a good fast pace and heart rate throughout

Step aerobics involves choreographed moves over and onto a platform or step, and work on both stamina and muscle conditioning. The height of the platform can be raised or lowered depending on how rigorous you want your workout to be. Step routines sometimes involve complex movements and dance steps, requiring good co-ordination. They can be good for toning up the muscles in the legs and backside, while the energy use and heart rates are similar to aerobics

Water-based aerobics derive their benefits from water resistance as well as water support and are a great class choice for people who are overweight, nursing an injury or elderly, because there's less stress placed on joints. Since the body is naturally buoyant in water momentum is eliminated, making it possible to work opposing muscle groups much more easily. Classes often use specially designed flotation and resistance devices, dumbbells and webbed gloves, or even high-density plastic steps that sit on the bottom of the pool. The coolness of the pool water can make exercise much more comfortable, especially if you're the type that overheats easily, and the support of the water makes stretching in a standing position much easier. Typically, you would work at 70-80% of your maximum heart rate using about 6 calories per minute.

Body conditioning/sculpting/toning classes usually begin with an aerobic warm-up followed by a range of exercises to tone, reshape and strengthen the muscles. Bodybars, elastic bands, Exertubes, hand and ankle weights are used to add resistance to the exercise. More recent additions to the muscle conditioning type of class include those using a large air-filled ball (such as a Swiss ball or a Flexaball) or Reebok Core Trainer, a flat board sitting on a moveable base (similar to a wobble board). Both devices are used as props with which to do a range of innovative exercises set to music.

OTHER CLASS TYPES

A range of other class types may also be available to you depending on the type of gym or health club you have access to. These are often considered to be more vigorous in intensity but less dance-based in the type of moves used in the aerobic and similar type classes outlined previously. The most popular ones include:

- studio cycling/spinning
- tae bo/khai bo/kick boxing
- boxercise
- circuits
- body pump

Studio cycling could be likened to aerobics on bikes. Classes are set to motivating music as participants ride specially designed stationary bikes on an imaginary journey over different terrain. Difficulty is varied by adjusting the tension knob and/or speed, which allows participants to climb hills, ride on a flat road, or fly downhill, in or out of the saddle. Best suited for an intermediate to advanced exerciser, studio cycling can provide an extremely vigorous and intense workout with little or no impact.

Circuit training, in all its varied forms, is athletic in nature so it's great for someone who's in reasonable physical condition, wants to be physically challenged, but doesn't want to think about following an intricate routine. The format usually involves alternating 'stations' of aerobic-type exercises (skipping, jumping-jacks, shuttle-runs) interspersed with conditioning-type exercises (push-ups, crunches and squats). Although the heart rate goes up and down, according to the exercise, the average heart rate should remain quite high throughout, but it relies on you pushing yourself hard enough.

Boxercise is a variation of circuit classes, which also includes a range of upper-body boxing moves. Classes require a reasonable level of agility, fitness and speed. Class formats frequently include an aerobic warm-up with continuous boxing moves and steps followed by circuit stations combining some punches using punch bags and gloves.

Tai Bo/Khai Bo/Cardio Kick Boxing incorporate a range of classes that have their roots in martial arts and can provide a safe and satisfying way to release stress – and even aggression, as you release punches and kicks. All are reasonably athletic and most routines are fundamentally basic in structure, utilising kicks, jabs, undercuts and uppercuts as core movements. As an intense total body workout, they all build upper body, legs, speed, endurance, timing and overall conditioning. The more advanced the class, the more intense the workout, but no matter what level you train at, you'll avoid injury and prevent painful hamstring pulls by never kicking above hip level.

Body Pump is basically weight training routines set to music and provides a great alternative to those who need the motivation or find resistance training on machines boring. Using a bar with plate weights and a step, each song focuses on a different muscle where the moves follow the beat of the music. Repetitions are high and you need to vary and increase the weight you put on the bar as you progress. These classes are great for toning and even building muscle depending on the amount of weight used, but would not be very effective in increasing stamina.

MORE RELAXING CLASS CHOICES

Many leisure centres now offer classes in stretch-based exercises such as Yoga, Tai Chi and Pilates. These are becoming more and more popular as a more relaxed mind-body approach to exercise and as a way of unwinding from our increasingly stressful lifestyles. In these classes, the emphasis is on relaxation and listening to the body, and may be done with very gentle or no music, and in a very calm and peaceful atmosphere. The most popular classes include:

- yoga
- pilates
- tai chi

Yoga is one of the most popular forms of relaxation exercise. The word yoga means 'union'. Yoga postures are said to unify the mind, body and breath so that they work together as one. There are many different types of Yoga but most use slow, controlled movements to stretch and tone the body, as in Hatha Yoga. Asthanga Yoga, although based on the same movements, is more vigorous and power-based in its moves. Either form is associated with inducing a feeling of well-being and relaxation, as well as improving posture and tone in areas such as the stomach, bottom and thighs.

Pilates is another form of relaxation exercise where the emphasis is on strengthening, realigning and balancing the body so that it performs in complete harmony. It teaches good breathing techniques, and makes participants more aware of their own body through a series of slow, controlled movements. Core strength around the abdominal area is a major focus as the way to control all movements. Pilates can be very effective in improving posture, movement and muscle tone and again it is suitable for people of all ages and all levels of fitness.

Tai Chi is an ancient Chinese technique based on the balance of energies that flow through the body. It is often referred to as 'Meditation in Motion' as it aims to promote a spiritual tranquillity along with increased mental and physical energy. Tai Chi consists of slow, flowing movements to relax the mind and body. Like Yoga, the emphasis is on performing all the exercises slowly and gently. Once you get to know the moves you are encouraged to do them as regularly on your own as a form of relaxation. Tai Chi can be effective in improving balance, posture and co-ordination and is suitable for people of all ages and all levels of fitness.

WHICH CLASS?

Your choice of class depends largely on what is available locally and then what you feel you might enjoy. After that, is a matter of deciding what your focus is – general fitness or posture or muscle tone – and matching a class with your level of fitness. Choosing a variety of classes is not a bad option to begin with until you find which ones you will stick with. If starting off, do a maximum of three classes a week. In your weekly exercise routine, it is often best to supplement class exercises with alternative, less structured activity such as brisk walking, cycling, swimming or running. If any of these can be outdoors, so much the better. This will give a better balance and the more muscles you involve in a range of different activities, the more effective your programme will be, and the less likely you are to develop an overuse injury.

Safety tips

- To minimize risk to your knees, keep your foot and knee aligned in the same direction with the knee directly above the foot when flexed.
- Always make sure that you warm up and cool down.
- Avoid any hyperextension of your back.
- Be aware of your posture – you should have your shoulders back and relaxed, tummy pulled in, hips forward.
- Never lock your knees straight: keep them slightly bent and 'soft' (relaxed).
- Do not go too deep or low if you are doing anything in a lunge or squat position.

WHAT TO WEAR

Wear any type of clothing that you feel most comfortable in. Cotton and nylon mixes are good as they are for sweat-absorbing. Lycra and some of the newer materials are also effective and comfortable. Loose clothing may be more appropriate for the relaxation-based classes. Shoes are your most important piece of equipment. Ideally you need a proper pair of indoor trainers – often called cross-trainers and either the boot or shoe type is fine, depending on which feels more comfortable. Make sure that they do not rub or irritate your Achilles tendon at the back of your ankle. The sole should be flexible and have good shock absorption and cushioning.

CHAPTER 11

Nutrition, Pills and Potions

There is a wealth of information, both good and bad, on sports nutrition, eating for health and slimming diets. Numerous nutritional supplements, pills, potions and other dietary aids are available, claiming to make improvements on performance, health or body shape.

A BALANCED DIET

Of course, there are no 'miracle' dietary supplements that will enable the average marathon runner to break the world record or an overweight person to shed 4 kilos in 2 weeks. The words 'balanced', 'nutritional' and 'healthy' used in the context of diet describe the way you should aim to eat – whether as a recreational or world-class competitor. A good, basic and well-balanced diet is critical for everyone, not only to fulfil your basic energy requirements but also to keep your whole body working efficiently.

Total energy intake

Carbohydrate, fat, protein and alcohol together make up your 'total energy intake' measured in *kilocalories* (the amount of heat released when these foods are broken down in your body). When fully broken down these nutrients release differing amounts of energy per gramme (a tiny amount). They are:

carbohydrate	4 kcals
fat	9 kcals
protein	4 kcals
alcohol	7 kcals

Ideal diet

Fat has twice the number of kilocalories per gramme compared to protein or carbohydrate. The ideal diet for fitness or for health should be biased towards a high proportion of carbohydrate and a low amount of fat, with adequate protein and fibre, and plenty of fluid. Unfortunately, the average Western diet is high in fat and alcohol and relatively low in carbohydrates and fibre.

Breakdown of an ideal diet

Whether you want to lose or gain or maintain weight, the same basic nutritional guidelines apply – only the amounts vary. You should aim to get:

- at least 50-60% of your energy from carbohydrate
- no more than 30-35% from fat
- about 12-15% from protein
- less than 4% from alcohol – yes, there is still a little room for alcohol in a healthy diet.

Carbohydrate

Cakes, sweets, sugary drinks, chocolate bars and so on are sources of carbohydrate (and fat). But these *simple* carbohydrates provide only sugar which gives you a quick energy boost and little else – after 1 biscuit, chocolate or sugary drink you need another to reboost your sugar levels. The more filling, starchy, *complex* carbohydrates (the type found in potatoes, rice, pasta, bread as well as in vegetables and pulses) provide energy *and* vitamins, minerals and fibre. Energy from these is released more slowly into the blood, enabling your body to maintain a *balanced* blood-sugar level (through the action of insulin). After the intake of such carbohydrates blood-sugar level may even be the same as before but you feel better.

Fat

Most of us eat more fat than we need, either knowingly or otherwise. Pastry has large amounts of hidden fat, mainly in the form of butter. The healthiest fats to eat are the (mainly) liquid *polyunsaturated fats*. These come from grain, seeds, vegetables, fruit and fish. *Saturated fats* come mainly from animal sources and tend to be more solid. Although both types have the same amount of kilocalories per given weight, saturated fats are more likely to lead to an increase in blood-cholesterol level, which is associated with increased risks of heart disease and other related illnesses. *Monounsaturated fats*, found in olive oil and nuts, are also a healthy choice and help to lower cholesterol.

Cholesterol
Cholesterol is a fat-like substance produced in many animal bodies. Animal foods such as egg yolks, shellfish, offal, cream and cheese are rich sources of cholesterol whereas vegetables tend to contain very little. Cholesterol is important to us for normal metabolism but our own bodies can produce the required quantity.

Protein
An adequate intake of protein is needed to build and repair muscle tissue, grow hair and fingernails, produce hormones and boost the immune system. Most sports people who eat moderate portions of protein-rich foods daily probably get more than they need. Any extra protein can be used as energy when carbohydrate stores are low, or it can be stored as fat. Red meat, traditionally regarded as the best source of protein, has the disadvantage of containing fat. White meat, fish and vegetables (such as pulses) are therefore preferable sources of protein.

Vitamins and minerals
A good, well-balanced diet should contain all the vitamins and minerals your body needs. You may additionally take a *multivitamin* supplement but be aware that there is no proven advantage to taking *individual* vitamin supplements.

FLUIDS

Sweating

Sweating enables your body to get rid of extra heat generated from muscle activity during exercise. If you are prone to heavy sweating it does not mean that you are unfit: it merely indicates that you generate considerable muscle heat. More problematic would be a lack of sweat as this could lead to overheating. If you drink too little or lose a lot of water through profuse sweating you will not be training or competing at your best. It is vital, therefore, to replace these fluids by drinking regularly. Pure water is to be preferred, but other drinks are useful too.

How much do you need to drink?

Weigh yourself before and after exercise in the same clothes. The difference in weight is the amount of fluid you have lost and need to replace. This is the amount of water that you need to drink:

1 kilogramme (2 lbs) weight loss = 1 litre (2 pints) of water to drink

Remember, this is in addition to your *normal* daily intake of fluid which should be about 2 litres or about 8 glasses of water. Fruit juices, drinks and soda (diet and regular) are acceptable, but water or low-sugar cordials are preferable. Tea and coffee are not ideal as they contain caffeine, which is a diuretic.

> A diuretic stimulates your body to lose more fluid. A sure way to become dehydrated is to drink excessive cups of tea or coffee after your training. Signs of dehydration include fatigue, headaches, dizziness and lethargy.

The urine colour test

A quick way to check if you are drinking enough is to examine the colour of your urine. If, shortly after exercise, the sample is dark in colour and small in amount, then you need to drink more. Urine is normally a pale yellow colour when you are adequately hydrated.

Drink while exercising

Get into the habit of drinking small amounts while you are exercising, particularly if it is hot or you continue for more than an hour. Aim to have about a cup (100 ml) every 15 minutes. If you are in the gym, take sips from the water cooler (if one is available). If you are outdoors, make sure you have a drinks bottle with you and take regular sips.

Sports drinks

Sports drinks contain varying amounts of carbohydrate and are formulated to be drunk before, during or after exercise. During exercise you should dilute the drink (that is, its sugar level) as concentrated drinks draw the blood and fluid away from muscles towards the digestive system. This will affect your exercise ability. After the activity you can drink a more concentrated drink to replace the energy and fluid.

Thirst is not a good indicator of when you need to drink, so drink before you are thirsty.

Alcohol

Alcohol is also a diuretic and can have a dehydrating effect (you take more trips to the toilet when drinking alcohol). It is not an effective way to rehydrate after a game. Also, in a can of beer only 50 of the total 150 kilocalories are from carbohydrate; the rest are alcohol. Alcohol is not converted to the energy type of carbohydrate stored in muscles (glycogen). Unfortunately, it is stored as fat.

GOOD HABITS

Timing

- Naturally, you should not eat just prior to exercise. Leave 2-3 hours after a meal before you exercise, particularly if the meal contains protein.
- If you have a good, healthy, high-carbohydrate diet, your muscles should be adequately fuelled for exercise.
- For a quick energy boost, or if you are training in the early evening and need something mid-afternoon, a light carbohydrate snack such as a banana, rice cake, slice of bread and honey, or bagel is ideal.
- Remember that high-calorie meals take longer to leave your stomach than lighter snacks. It is best not to have sugary foods up to 30 minutes before exercise as these can lead to a drop in your blood-sugar level.

Refuelling your muscles

The first hour after you finish your training or match is the most important time to refuel your muscles. Immediately after exercise your metabolic rate is high and your muscles' ability to replenish those vital glycogen stores is at its peak. If you don't feel like eating immediately after exercise, drink a sugary drink or fruit juice, or try to eat a banana. These provide carbohydrate to start the refuelling wheels in motion. If you have done a particularly strenuous training session or played a hard game, lasting over an hour, your carbohydrate stores will be almost completely empty. It can take 24-48 hours to refill these stores (and that is on a good diet). The sooner you start this recovery the better, particularly if you are training again the next day.

Improving your nutrition

Step 1
Increase your carbohydrate intake.

- Pasta, rice, bread, potatoes, cereals and noodles should be the biggest part of your diet.
- Make sandwiches with thicker slices of bread and use less filling.
- Add pasta or rice to salads and dried fruit to cereals or yoghurt.
- Pizza bases are great but go easy on the cheese and pile up with vegetable topping.

Below is a list of sources of carbohydrates. As we explained earlier in the chapter, the best sources are complex carbohydrates but simple carbohydrates are useful for a quick energy boost.

Sources of Carbohydrates

- breakfast cereals – include some wholegrain varieties
- bread – all types, e.g. wholemeal, granary, white soft grain, white bread, pitta bread, french bread, rolls, baps, muffins, crumpets, bagels and potato cakes
- crispbread, water biscuits, wholemeal crackers, oatcakes and rice cakes
- pasta – all shapes and colours
- rice
- potatoes – boiled, mashed and jacket more often than chips, roast or crisps
- popcorn and sweetcorn
- pizza bases – deep pan (care with the topping)
- beans – baked, red kidney, borlotti
- peas, lentils, chickpeas and pearl barley
- root vegetables – carrots, parsnips, swedes, beetroot

If you are exercising for more than an hour and a half, you will find it helpful to drink during exercise fluid which contains some sugar. Ensure the drink-container label states that the carbohydrate content is no more than 8%.

- fruit – all sorts, fresh, dried or canned
- fruit juice
- natural or fruit yoghurt
- cereal bars (be careful about the fat content)
- jam, marmalade, honey, syrup and treacle
- confectionery
- biscuits – Rich Tea, Nice, fig roll, plain digestives rather than shortbread or custard creams because of the fat content
- cakes – currant buns, malt or fruit loaf, fruit cakes, scones, gingerbread, parkin, rock cakes and other similar 'simple or plain' cakes. Go easy on others which may have high fat content
- puddings – fruit crumbles, baked fruit, bread pudding, milk puddings, jelly or banana custard
- sweetened soft drinks and flavoured milk drinks
- sugar – added to drinks and breakfast cereals
- sports products, e.g. glucose polymer drinks.

Step 2
Keep an eye on the amount of fat you eat.

- Grill, boil, steam or microwave meat, fish or poultry rather than fry.
- Choose lean cuts of meat and trim off extra fat.
- Choose chicken or fish rather than red meat.
- Cut down on all fried foods, especially prepared pies, chips and crisps.
- Choose low-fat cheese, butter, margarine, milk and yoghurt. Lower-fat cheeses include Edam, Camembert, Brie, mozzarella, feta or cottage cheese.
- Add less of a strong cheese, such as Gruyère or Gouda, to sauces.
- Use less oil in cooking and cook in a non-stick pan.
- Choose low-fat or tomato-based sauces rather than cream sauces on pasta, rice or meat.

Step 3
Choose healthy snacks:

- bagels, rice cakes, oatcakes, English muffins, crumpets, bread, rolls, pitta bread or crackers with jam, honey or Marmite
- dried and fresh fruits, especially bananas
- fruit juice and soft drinks
- yoghurt and popcorn
- breakfast cereals with skimmed milk
- muesli bars, but watch out for fat.

Step 4

Eat regularly and do not skip any meals (especially breakfast).

Step 5

Drink plenty of water and other fluids.

- Drink at least 2-3 litres of water per day.
- Get into the habit of carrying a water bottle with you.

Step 6

Start the refuelling process in the first hour after exercise.

- Not hungry? Drink some fruit juice.

Step 7

- Avoid eating late at night.

MANAGING YOUR BODY FAT AND WEIGHT

EXERCISE AND FAT LOSS

Whilst exercise has an important role to play in maintaining a healthy body weight, and more importantly, a healthy body fat level, we can never ignore the food side of the equation. Putting a huge effort into your exercise regime whilst eating excessive amounts of the wrong foods is a sure-fire way of upsetting the balance and eventually gaining weight and body fat. It really just negates all the hard work of exercise. However, if you have gained weight or become out of shape for whatever reason, what is the best way to deal with it?

Eating for fat loss depends not just on the amount you eat and drink, but also on the what and when. The trick is in learning to eat and drink what your body needs and avoid what it doesn't need. The most effective way to reduce body fat is through creating a deficit or imbalance of at least 300 kcals per day, but preferably closer to 500 kcals. It is much easier to do this through a reduction of calorie intake (of 150 – 250 kcals) combined with an increase in energy expenditure by the same amount through exercise.

A reduction of 150 kcals might be eating one less slice of bread, butter and jam, 2 less biscuits, one less glass of wine or pint of beer on a daily basis. A reduction in 250 kcals might entail cutting out that slice of cake/bar of chocolate, biscuit and hot chocolate or 2 slices of toast and butter. An increase in exercise equivalent to 150 - 200 calories could be a brisk 30-minute walk, a 15-minute jog or a 20-minute continuous swim. You can check out the energy burned up in different activities for your body weight in Appendix 3.

Creating a deficit of just 300 kcals per day would amount to the equivalent of 20 lbs of fat loss in a year!

The simplest method is to choose a routine, whether eating or exercise, that can become a habit rather than a short term change for a fixed period. Of course, we all need to set goals, which might be getting in shape for a certain event or occasion, and this is a good way to maintain the motivation to introduce some new changes. Once a new healthier eating pattern has become manageable and habitual, it is time to introduce a few more changes such as cutting down on fat by taking a close look at all the ways it may creep into your daily eating pattern. How about deciding to take on two new healthier habits every 3 or 4 weeks? Once each one becomes a habit, introduce a new one. Add to this a gradual increase in either pace, duration or choice of activities and you will be well on your way to a leaner you.

Another factor in weight management is eating regularly. Meal skipping and leaving long gaps between meals is an almost guaranteed way to gain body fat. The long gaps without food or nourishment send the body into 'starvation' or 'conservation' mode, as it slows down the metabolic rate to conserve energy, in case there is no input for a prolonged period. If this happens regularly, the metabolism just adapts to a slower rate and you need fewer calories in the day. In addition, after a long gap without eating, we tend to reach for higher fat or sugar foods that give an instant or more satisfying energy boost, rather than a more healthy lower fat or sugar option that the body actually needs. Add to this the fact that, when we do eat after a long gap, the body will preferentially store it as fat, just in case another long gap lies ahead.

YOU AND YOUR BODY SHAPE

It is worth pointing out at this stage that successful, long-term weight management does depend partly on the body type and shape that you have genetically inherited, and partly on maintaining a relative amount of lean or muscle tissue. Although we cannot change the genetic part, we can certainly do a lot to maintain and keep our muscle active through exercise.

Body types are commonly described in three broad categories:

- the taller, angular, lean type
- the moderate height, muscular type
- the shorter, more curvy, broader hips type

However, many of us fall in between two categories, having characteristics of both. The point about knowing your body type is accepting it, especially with respect to setting your goals. But, no matter what your body type you will always have the capacity to maintain and activate your muscle. The difference is that some individuals tend to gain muscle more easily than others, which is dependent on their basic body type. Since each kilogram of muscle burns up 110 calories per day compared with about 5 calories per day for each kg of fat, you can see the reason to increase the amount of muscle you have. This does not mean developing large muscles; merely activating and improving the function and condition of what is already there (but often hidden) is sufficient. Naturally, increasing the amount of muscle is more effective, since any increase in muscle will lead to an increase in metabolism, leading ultimately to a decrease in body fat.

This is the reason that dieting alone is not usually effective in the long term, as the metabolism gradually adapts to a new daily energy requirement and your body will just learn to survive on fewer calories. Add exercise, and muscle conditioning/strengthening exercises in particular, and you not only prevent the decrease in metabolic rate, but you can actually speed it up.

The bottom line: healthy eating and appropriate activity, including muscle-conditioning exercises, will mean long-term attainment of a healthy body fat and shape which is easier to maintain.

CALCULATING YOUR ENERGY REQUIREMENTS

The amount of calories you need to eat in a day is a very individual requirement, which is influenced by your current weight, body composition and body type. Your daily calorie requirement is determined by:

1. your basic metabolic rate (BMR)
2. your lifestyle
3. your digestion
4. your activity levels

1. Your individual BMR is the calories your body needs when you are at rest (or sitting all day) and can be calculated from the formula below:

MEN
66.5 + (13.75 x your weight in kg) + (5 x height in cm) – (6.75 x age in yrs)

WOMEN
665 + (9.55 x your weight in kg) + (1.8 x height in cm) – (4.7 x age in yrs)

2. Your lifestyle adds an extra percentage to your BMR depending on your daily occupation excluding activity. If you have a :

- sedentary lifestyle (office work, teaching, student): add 20% to your BMR
- moderately active lifestyle (housewife, salesperson, teacher): add 40% to your BMR
- very active lifestyle (manual worker): add 80% to your BMR

3. Add another 200 calories to account for the calories used up in digestion of the food you eat during the day.
4. You can work out the number of calories used up in any activities you do, according to your body weight, using the chart in Appendix 2.

Add the four figures together to get you own individual daily calorie requirement

EXAMPLE
Jane is 28 years old, works full time in a bank, and runs for 45 minutes (5 miles) most evenings after work. Her height is 168cm and weight is 60kg. Her BMR is calculated from:

$$665 + (9.55 \times 60) + (1.8 \times 168) - (4.7 \times 28) = 1399 \text{ calories} => \textbf{1400 calories}$$

Multiply this by 20% to account for her job/lifestyle expenditure (1400 x 0.2 = 280) and add it on plus add on the 200 calories for daily digestion:

Jane's BMR is 1400 + 280 + 200 = **1880 calories per day**

Her daily run would burn up 12 calories per min x 45 mins = **540 calories**

Therefore Jane's daily energy requirement would be **2420 CALORIES**

DECODING THE FOOD LABEL

How may of us continually look at labels on any food items we buy? Do you know what it all means or what you are looking at? Labels vary considerably in how much and what type of information they give, and the wording used can be confusing and even misleading, as can the pictures. It could add hours onto your shopping if you tried to decipher all the information given on the range of products you buy.

Here is a quick summary of the main parts of the label that you should be aware of, plus a guide to what you need of the main ingredients on a daily basis.

WHAT'S IN THE LABEL?

Nutritional claim	What it means
Low calorie	No more than 40 calories in a normal serving
Reduce calorie/fat/ sugar/sodium	At least 25% fewer claories than a standard version of the same food
Low fat	Less than 5g in a normal serving
Low sugar	Less than 5g in a normal serving
Low salt	Less than 40g in a normal serving
High fibre	At least 6g of fibre in 100g of the food

HOW MUCH DO WE NEED?

Per 100g

	A lot means	A little means
Sugars	10g or more	2g or less
Fats	15g or more	3g or less
Saturates	5g or more	1g or less
Fibre	3g or more	0.5g or less
Sodium	0.5g or more	0.1g or less

DAILY RECOMMENDED INTAKE

	Men	Women
Sugars	Up to 70g	Up to 50g
Fats	Up to 95g	Up to 70g
Saturates	Up to 30g	Up to 20g
Fibre	At Least 20g	At Least 16g
Sodium	Up to 2.5g	Up to 2g
Protein	About 65-75g	About 55-65g

CHAPTER 12

Coping with Injury

Being fit and active and taking part in sport are good for you in very many ways. However, risk of injury cannot be ignored. Professional sportsmen and women are, unfortunately, regularly forced to stop playing due to injury. You yourself may have been put out of action through injury at some stage in your sporting career.

AVOIDING INJURY

You can reduce the risk of sustaining an injury if you follow these general guidelines:

- Use a well-planned exercise programme.
- Be patient and progress gradually.
- Ensure you have the right footwear and equipment.
- Train on a suitable, safe surface.

Here are a few essential steps that will prevent, or at least reduce, the risk of injury whether you are starting off, resuming a training programme, or already reasonably fit and training hard.

Warming up

A warm-up allows you to adapt gradually to the demands of exercise by raising your body's temperature. This in turn increases the pliability of the muscles and ligaments, boosts the circulation and diverts the blood flow to where it is required (see Chapters 1 and 7 for more details on warming up). At the gym, any properly run exercise class will include a warm-up.

Begin a warm-up with a gentle, whole-body activity.

- Brisk walking or jogging, or marching or jogging on the spot while also rotating the shoulders and swinging the arms to loosen them up, are good exercises.
- If you are swimming, start off with some arm circling and shoulder rotating out of the water followed by 5 minutes of *gentle* swimming before you start to swim properly.
- Follow this gentle, whole-body activity with some stretching exercises but don't force the stretches at this stage. Stretching is more effective *after* exercise when the body is fully warmed up.

> It is always tempting to go straight on to a court or a pitch and start playing tennis, squash, badminton, football, hockey and so on. This is looking for trouble. Warming up is particularly important in sports that involve much twisting, turning and reaching, all of which can easily strain or pull a cold muscle.

Cooling down

Leave time for a cool-down at the end of your training session. The reverse of the warm-up process, a cool-down allows the body temperature to decrease and the circulation to return gradually to normal. This prevents the build-up ('pooling') of blood and the waste products of exercise in the muscles. A good cool-down can work wonders in preventing post-exercise aches and stiffness. (See Chapter 1 for more details on cooling down.)

- Slow down gradually from whatever activity you were doing and then walk or jog slowly for a few minutes.
- Follow this with some stretching exercises, concentrating particularly on the muscles you have used.

Footwear and equipment

In most activities the feet take first impact, and the weight going through your foot can be at least 3 times your body weight. So look after your feet with shoes that fit well. There is no point in buying a pair of tennis shoes if you plan to take up jogging, and don't try and get

> If you are exercising outdoors at night, wear reflective clothing. If it is very cold wear numerous thin layers to trap the air. Putting Vaseline on the lips and exposed areas also protects from the cold.

away with an old pair of shoes that have been gathering dust in a cupboard for years. Well-cushioned shoes absorb a lot of the surface impact shock and protect the knee joints and the back. Choose appropriate shoes for your main activity, bearing in mind the surface and the location (indoors or outdoors). If unsure, ask for advice. Also, use appropriate protective equipment. For example:

- knee pads in volleyball
- shin guards in hockey and football
- gum shields in rugby
- safety helmets in cycling.

Avoid overheating and hypothermia

If exercising in very warm temperatures, remember that the body still needs to warm up and you must drink plenty of fluids. In cold weather even though you sweat less you must still drink plenty of fluids. If you are exercising in very cold temperatures, prepare well by wearing several layers. Hypothermia, the opposite of overheating, is most frequently seen in climbers.

Vary the surface

Try not to do all your training on the same type of surface. For example, if you do a lot of running, vary the surface between grass, roads, tracks and treadmill. This helps to avoid over-stressing a particular muscle group, tendon or ligament, and also leads to a better all-round adaptation.

Listen to your body

Don't exercise if you are feeling under the weather or have a heavy cold. This will put undue stress on the body and will cause you to tire earlier. It could also lead to a more serious illness from a relatively minor infection.

Progress gradually

A sure way to increase your injury risk is to increase your training volume, distance or intensity too quickly. Pace your progression and don't rush it!

Effective physical preparation

Injuries can also be prevented through effective preparation, both skills- and fitness-wise. Skilful players are less likely to get injured as they are usually ahead of the game and can avoid dangerous moves or tackles. This skill is developed mainly through adequate practice. Adequate physical preparation will give you the right amount of flexibility, stamina and strength to match the demands of your sport so that you are not forced to push yourself beyond your ability.

ARE YOU INJURED?

You have taken all the necessary precautions but you still have a niggling pain in your calf/hip. How do you know if you have a sports injury, and what should you do?

Muscles, tendons and ligaments

The majority of minor sports injuries are due to damage to muscles, ligaments and tendons rather than fractures and broken bones.

- Muscle strain results when muscle fibres are overstretched or torn.
- Tendons, which join muscles to bones, can become inflamed or torn when overused. For example, the Achilles tendon above the heel can become sore through using inappropriate footwear or too much exercise on the wrong surface.
- Ligaments, which join bones together at the joints, can be strained, torn or ruptured through sudden movements, turns, falls or twists. It is usually a ligament that is damaged when you go over on your ankle or twist the knee outwards in a sudden change of direction.

These most common injuries frequently begin with a niggling or dull pain in a specific area. This is not to be confused with normal muscle ache (felt after a new activity or exercise), which lasts about 4 days. Pains lasting longer than a week may be more serious. Strained muscles and ligaments frequently result in local swelling, redness and a warm feeling in the area. Some of these types of injury will disappear after a few weeks if you decrease the amount of activity you are doing or change to another activity that does not stress the same area. Or try simply changing your footwear.

Self-treatment steps

For any muscle or ligament strain or pull there are a few simple self-treatment steps you should always follow. The acronym RICE will help you remember these:

1. **R**est – take the weight off the injured area and rest it as much as possible.
2. **I**ce – use it to reduce swelling and pain. Keep the ice pack on for 10-15 minutes at a time until your skin turns red.
3. **C**ompression – use a bandage or broad-width strapping to reduce swelling and potentially reduce the effect of an injury. Remove strapping every 4-5 hours and when sleeping.
4. **E**levation – raise the injured limb to encourage blood flow away from the arca and reduce swelling.

By taking these steps and allowing a gradual build-up to your previous level of activity you will avoid a more serious injury that would require specific treatment. However, if pain persists, seek appropriate advice.

Don't take risks. If the injury persists, stop exercising and seek professional advice.

Appendix 1: Records

Weekly Training Schedule

This schedule allows you to keep a bi-monthly record of what you did in your training each day. It should be a broad description. The details of your schedule should be noted in resistance-training and aerobic-training records.

Week 1	a.m.	p.m.
Mon	run	
Tues	rest	weights
Wed	weights	
Thurs	—	speed work
Fri	—	run
Sat	tennis	weights
Sun	rest	—

Week 1	a.m.	p.m.
Mon		
Tues		
Wed		
Thurs		
Fri		
Sat		
Sun		

Week 2	a.m.	p.m.
Mon		
Tues		
Wed		
Thurs		
Fri		
Sat		
Sun		

continued

Week 3	a.m.	p.m.
Mon		
Tues		
Wed		
Thurs		
Fri		
Sat		
Sun		

Week 4	a.m.	p.m.
Mon		
Tues		
Wed		
Thurs		
Fri		
Sat		
Sun		

Week 5	a.m.	p.m.
Mon		
Tues		
Wed		
Thurs		
Fri		
Sat		
Sun		

Week 6	a.m.	p.m.
Mon		
Tues		
Wed		
Thurs		
Fri		
Sat		
Sun		

Week 7	a.m.	p.m.
Mon		
Tues		
Wed		
Thurs		
Fri		
Sat		
Sun		

Week 8	a.m.	p.m.
Mon		
Tues		
Wed		
Thurs		
Fri		
Sat		
Sun		

Aerobic Training Record

Record the mode of training, the intensity of the session, the duration of the session and pertinent notes on conditions, how you felt, etc.

Name: _____ DOB: _____

Sport: _____ Position: _____ Club: _____

Period: ☐ foundation (base)   ☐ pre-season   ☐ in-season

MHR: ☐ 60% MHR   ☐ 75% MHR   ☐ 80% MHR

Date	Mode	Intensity (% of MHR)	Training heart-rate range (bpm)	Duration of session (min)

Key: use the following symbols to help describe your sessions:

——	steady pace		windy
~	varied pace/intensity		cloudy
(sun)	sunny		cloudy and cool/cold
(H)	sunny and hot		rain

Distance covered/ reps done (as appropriate)	Notes

Resistance-training Record

Record the exercises, weights (wts), sets and reps you use. Indicate whether the training is in the foundation, pre-season or in-season period. Make additional notes as a narrative to your work.

Exercise	Date:	workout 1				workout 2			
1	Sets								
	Reps								
	Wts (kg)								
2	Sets								
	Reps								
	Wts (kg)								
3	Sets	w/u	1	2	3•	1	2•	3	4•
	Reps	15	12	10	10	10	10	10	8
	Wts (kg)	50	90	110	120	110	120	130	130
4	Sets								
	Reps								
	Wts (kg)								
5	Sets								
	Reps								
	Wts (kg)								
6	Sets								
	Reps								
	Wts (kg)								
7	Sets								
	Reps								
	Wts (kg)								

Name: _____ DOB: _____

Sport: _____ Position: _____ Club: _____

Period: ☐ foundation (base) ☐ pre-season ☐ in-season

MHR: ☐ 60% MHR ☐ 75% MHR ☐ 80% MHR

workout 3   *workout 4*

Notes

☺ especially in set 2
IRM = 140 on 17/6
diet going especially well

continued

245

Resistance-training Record (continued)

Name: _____ DOB: _____

Sport: _____ Position: _____ Club: _____

Period: ☐ foundation (base) ☐ pre-season ☐ in-season

MHR: ☐ 60% MHR ☐ 75% MHR ☐ 80% MHR

Exercise	Date:	*workout 5*				*workout 6*			
1	Sets								
	Reps								
	Wts (kg)								
2	Sets								
	Reps								
	Wts (kg)								
3	Sets								
	Reps								
	Wts (kg)								
4	Sets								
	Reps								
	Wts (kg)								
5	Sets								
	Reps								
	Wts (kg)								
6	Sets								
	Reps								
	Wts (kg)								
7	Sets								
	Reps								
	Wts (kg)								

Key: use the following symbols as appropriate:

w/u warm-up set

• worked to failure, could only just
  manage/not manage this weight

IRM= one rep max weight (note weight achieved/date)

☺ Good session, worked well

☺ OK session, could have
  pushed harder

☹ Poor session (note reasons)

workout 7   *workout 8*

Notes

Appendix 2

Energy Expenditure

Portions of food containing approx. 50 grams carbohydrate

Fruit

Semi-dried mixed fruit	250-g pack
Dried apricots	125 g
Raisins	83 g
Pears	4-5 medium
Oranges	4-5 medium
Apples	4-5 medium
Bananas	3 medium
Tinned fruit in natural juice	410-g can

Vegetables

Baked potato	6-oz size
Parsnip	8-oz size
Instant Mash	60 g (half an average pack)

Breakfast cereals

Porridge (made with water)	2 average helpings*
Shredded Wheat	3½*
Weetabix	4 biscuits*

Kilocalories per minute expended for each activity

		Your body weight				
	kg	50	53	56	59	62
Activity	lb	110	117	123	130	137
Badminton						
leisure		4.9	5.1	5.4	5.7	6.0
tournament		7.3	7.7	8.1	8.6	9.0
Basketball						
competition		7.4	7.9	8.3	8.7	9.2
practice		6.9	7.3	7.7	8.1	8.6
Cycling						
leisure, 5.5 mph		3.2	3.4	3.6	3.8	4.0
leisure, 9.4 mph		5.0	5.3	5.6	5.9	6.2
racing, fast		8.5	9.0	9.5	10.0	10.5

| Alpen | 6 tablespoons* |
| Branflakes | 2 average helpings* |

* Quarter of a pint of low-fat milk will add another 6 g carbohydrate.

Bakery products

Fruit scones	1½
Chelsea bun	1⅓
Crumpets	3½
Pitta bread	1½ large size
White bap	1½
White bread	5 slices

Grains and cereals

Rice (uncooked)	75 g
Pasta (wholewheat, uncooked)	75 g
Pasta (white, uncooked)	70 g
Pizza base (thick)	½ × 22-cm base
Canned spaghetti in tomato sauce	¾ × 425-g can

| 65 | 68 | 71 | 74 | 77 | 80 | 83 | 86 | 89 | 92 |
143	150	157	163	170	176	183	190	196	203
6.3	6.6	6.9	7.2	7.5	7.8	8.1	8.3	8.6	8.9
9.4	9.9	10.4	10.8	11.2	11.6	12.1	12.5	12.9	13.4
9.6	10.1	10.5	10.9	11.4	11.8	12.3	12.7	13.1	13.6
9.0	9.4	9.8	10.2	10.6	11.0	11.5	11.9	12.3	12.7
4.2	4.4	4.5	4.7	4.9	5.1	5.3	5.5	5.7	5.9
6.5	6.8	7.1	7.4	7.7	8.0	8.3	8.6	8.9	9.2
11.0	11.5	12.0	12.5	13.0	13.5	14.0	14.5	15.0	15.5

continued

Kilocalories per minute expended for each activity (continued)

Activity	kg / lb	50 / 110	53 / 117	56 / 123	59 / 130	62 / 137
Field hockey			7.1	7.5	7.9	8.3
Football, competition			7.0	7.4	7.8	8.2
Golf		4.3	4.5	4.8	5.0	5.3
Racquetball		8.9	9.4	10.0	10.5	11.0
Running, on flat surface						
9 min per mile		9.7	10.2	10.8	11.4	12.0
7 min per mile			12.7	13.3	13.9	14.5
Skiing, soft snow						
leisure (female)		4.9	5.2	5.5	5.8	6.1
leisure (male)		5.6	5.9	6.2	6.5	6.9
Squash		10.6	11.2	11.9	12.5	13.1
Swimming, fitness swims						
backstroke		8.5	9.0	9.5	10.0	10.5
breaststroke		8.1	8.6	9.1	9.6	10.0
butterfly		8.6	9.1	9.6	10.1	10.7
crawl, fast		7.8	8.3	8.7	9.2	9.7
Tennis						
competition		7.3	7.8	8.2	8.7	9.1
recreational		5.5	5.8	6.1	6.4	6.8
Volleyball						
competition		7.3	7.8	8.2	8.7	9.1
recreational		2.5	2.7	2.8	3.0	3.1

Your body weight column headers: kg (50, 53, 56, 59, 62); lb (110, 117, 123, 130, 137)

65 143	68 150	71 157	74 163	77 170	80 176	83 183	86 190	89 196	92 203
8.7	9.1	9.5	9.9	10.3	10.7	11.1	11.5	11.9	12.3
8.6	9.0	9.4	9.8	10.2	10.6	11.0	11.4	11.7	12.1
5.5	5.8	6.0	6.3	6.5	6.8	7.1	7.3	7.6	7.8
11.6	12.1	12.6	13.2	13.7	14.2	14.8	15.3	15.8	16.4
12.5	13.1	13.7	14.3	14.9	15.4	16.0	16.6	17.2	17.8
15.0	15.6	16.2	16.8	17.4	17.9	18.5	19.1	19.7	20.3
6.4	6.7	7.0	7.3	7.5	7.8	8.1	8.4	8.7	9.0
7.2	7.5	7.9	8.2	8.5	8.9	9.2	9.5	9.9	10.2
13.8	14.4	15.1	15.7	16.3	17.0	17.6	18.2	18.9	19.5
11.0	11.5	12.0	12.5	13.0	13.5	14.0	14.5	15.0	15.5
10.5	11.0	11.5	12.0	12.5	13.0	13.4	13.9	14.4	14.9
11.1	11.7	12.2	12.7	13.2	13.7	14.2	14.2	15.2	15.8
10.1	10.6	11.1	11.5	12.0	12.5	12.9	13.4	13.9	14.4
9.5	9.9	10.2	10.6	11.1	11.5	11.9	12.4	12.8	13.2
7.1	7.4	7.7	8.1	8.4	8.7	9.0	9.4	9.7	10.0
9.5	10.0	10.5	10.9	11.4	11.8	12.3	12.7	13.1	13.6
3.3	3.4	3.6	3.7	3.9	4.0	4.2	4.3	4.5	4.6

Hillsborough College

Learning Resource Centre
Telephone: 0114 2602254

Appendix 3

The Muscular System

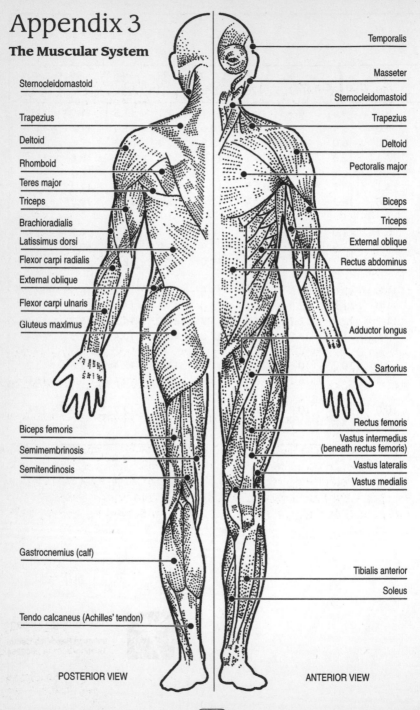

Sternocleidomastoid

Trapezius

Deltoid

Rhomboid

Teres major

Triceps

Brachioradialis

Latissimus dorsi

Flexor carpi radialis

External oblique

Flexor carpi ulnaris

Gluteus maximus

Biceps femoris

Semimembrinosis

Semitendinosis

Gastrocnemius (calf)

Tendo calcaneus (Achilles' tendon)

Temporalis

Masseter

Sternocleidomastoid

Trapezius

Deltoid

Pectoralis major

Biceps

Triceps

External oblique

Rectus abdominus

Adductor longus

Sartorius

Rectus femoris

Vastus intermedius
(beneath rectus femoris)

Vastus lateralis

Vastus medialis

Tibialis anterior

Soleus

POSTERIOR VIEW

ANTERIOR VIEW

Select Bibliography

Asterita, M.F., *Physical Exercise, Nutrition and Stress*, Praeger, New York, 1986.

Bean, Anita, *The Complete Guide to Sports Nutrition*, A. & C. Black, London, 1993.

Fahey, T.D., Insel, P.M., and Walton, T.R., *Fit and Well*, Mayfield, California, 1997.

Hockey, R.V., *Physical Fitness: the Pathway to Healthful Living*, Mosby, St. Louis, 1993.

Ratzin Jackson, C.G., *Nutrition for the Recreational Athlete*, CRC Series on Nutrition in Exercise and Sport.

Jones, G., and Hardy, L., eds, *Stress and Performance in Sport*, John Wiley & Sons Ltd, Chichester, 1990.

Katch, Frank I. and McCardle, William D., *Nutrition, Weight Control and Exercise*, Lea & Febiger, Philadelphia, 1988.

Ottaway, Peter Berry, and Hargin, Kevin, *Food for Sport: a Handbook of Sports Nutrition*, Resource Publications, Cambridge, 1985.

Wootton, Steve, *Nutrition for Sport*, Simon & Schuster, London, 1988.

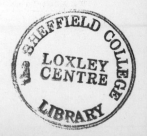
SHEFFIELD COLLEGE
LOXLEY CENTRE
LIBRARY

More information about nutrition for sport can be obtained from:

The Sports Nutrition Foundation
National Sports Medicine Institute
St Bartholomew's Medical College
Charterhouse Square
London EC1M 6BQ

Index